FOUNDATIONS OF HISTORY

Medicine Through Time

FIONA REYNOLDSON

Heinemann

Heinemann Library
Halley Court, Jordan Hill, Oxford OX2 8EJ
a division of Reed Educational &
Professional Publishing Ltd

OXFORD FLORENCE PRAGUE MADRID ATHENS
MELBOURNE AUCKLAND KUALA LUMPUR
SINGAPORE TOKYO IBADAN NAIROBI KAMPALA
JOHANNESBURG GABORONE PORTSMOUTH NH (USA)
CHICAGO MEXICO CITY SAO PAULO

© Fiona Reynoldson, 1996

First published 1996

Paperback edition published 1997

00 99 98 97 96
10 9 8 7 6 5 4 3 2 1

British Library Cataloguing in Publication Data
A catalogue record for this book is available from
the British Library

ISBN 0 431 05832 6 (0 431 05827 X PB) (614.09)

Produced by Dennis Fairey and Associates Ltd
Cover design by The Wooden Ark Studio
Illustrated by Arthur Phillips
Printed and Bound in Spain by Mateu Cromo

NOTE Some of the words and phrases printed in **bold** are
listed in the glossary on page 126.

Acknowledgements

The publishers would like to thank the following for permission to
reproduce copyright material:

Ancient Art and Architecture Collection: 1.1A, 5.3I Chester Beatty
Library, Dublin 7.4F Tim Beddow/Science Photo Library 12.3P
Count Robert Bégoüen, Musée Pujol, France: 1.2C Bodleian Library 8.4F
9.1A Bridgeman Art Library 2.2A British Library Reproductions 8.4G,
8.7O, 9T British Museum Library 4.6I, 9.2G Cambridge University
Library 8.2D Jean-Loup Charmet/Science Photo Library 11.4M
Coo.ee Historical Picture Archive 1.4E, 1.4F Corbis Bettmann/UPI
12.2L Francesca Countway Library 12.1C C. M. Dixon 3.1A, 3.2B,
4.1A, 5.3H E. T. Archive 4.6K, 12.1A Mary Evans Picture Library 10.1
(top box p.75), 11.1 (box p.79), 11.1C, 11.2I, 11.3 (box p. 83), 11.5
(box p.88), 12.5 (top box p. 108), 13.3(2) Alexander Fleming Laboratory
Museum, St Mary's Hospital, Paddington 11.5O, 11.5P Frank Graham
5.3G Hildesheim Museum 2.3C Michael Holford 4.3F, 5.3E, 7.2B Tim
Holt/Science Photo Library 12.3T Hulton Deutsch Collection 11.3J,
12,2 (box p.103), 12.5 (bottom box p.108), 13.2 (box p.112) Hutchinson
Library 12.3S Louvre Ager 4.7L Mansell Collection 10.1B, 12.4U, 13.1B,
13.2K Master and Fellows, Trinity College, Cambridge 8.6M Musee
Pasteur 11.3 (box p.83), 11.6(1) National Portrait Gallery, London 9
(p.72) Natural History Museum 12B Punch Library 13.2L, 13.2N,
13.2O Ann Ronan Picture Library 8.5I, 9.4Q Royal College of Surgeons
(bottom box p. 75), cover, 10.1A Science Photo Library 12.1G Ronald
Sheridan/Ancient Art and Architecture Collection 3E, 4.2D Paul Shuter
p.35 Topham Picture Library 12.3M University of Bradford,
Department of Archaeological Sciences, Calvin Wells Collection 1.2D
Wellcome Institute Library 2.5I, 4.2C, 7.3C, 7.6H, 12.1F, 12.2J, 12.4Z,
13.1C, 13,2E, 13.3(1) Werner Forman Archive 7.5G, 12.4X
West Stowe Country Park 6D Zentrale Farbbild Agentur 9.1B

Thanks are also due to *Health Which?* December 1992, published by
Consumers' Association, 2 Marylebone Rd, London NW1 4DF, for the
chart on page 120.

Details of written sources

In some sources the wording or sentence structure has been simplified
to ensure that the source is accessible.

Paul Addison, 'A New Jerusalem', in *Britain 1918-51*, Heinemann
Educational, 1994: 13.2M
Paul Addison, *Now the War is Over*, Cape, 1985: 13.2P, 13.2R
Michael Alexander, *Earliest English Poems*, Penguin, 1966: 6A
W.J. Bishop, *Early History of Surgery*, 1960: 7.4E
Marie Boas, *The Scientific Renaissance 1450-1630*, Penguin, 1972: 9.2C
Derrick Boxley, *Jenner and Smallpox Vaccine*, Heinemann, 1981:
11.1E, 11.1F
R.A. Browne, *British Latin Selections, AD 500-1400*, Blackwell, 1954: 8.7Y
J. Chadwick, W.N. Mann, I. M. Ionie & E.T. Withington, *Hippocratic
Writings*, Penguin, 1983: 4.3G, 4.8(2)
R. J. Cootes, *The Welfare State*, Longman, 1970: 13.2Q
Nancy Dunn & Dr Jenny Sutcliffe, *A History of Medicine From Prehistory
to the Year 2020*, Simon and Schuster, 1992: 12.1A
M. W. Flynn (ed.), *A Report of the Sanitary Conditions of the Labouring
Population of Great Britain*, Edinburgh University Press, 1965:
13.1F, 13.1H
GLC, *A History of the Black Presence in London*, GLC, 1986: 12.4W
H. L. Gordon, *Sir James Young Simpson and Chloroform*, 1897: 12.1E
W. A. Greenhill (trans.), *A Treatise on the Smallpox and Measles by Rhazes*,
Sydenham Society, 1848: 7.3D
Alastair McIntosh Gray, *Medical Care and Public Health: 1780 to the Present
Day*, OUP, 1990: 11.5Q, 11.5R
Douglas Guthrie, *A History of Medicine*, Nelson, 1945: 8.5J
Knut Haeger, *The Illustrated History of Surgery*, Harold Starke, 1988: 12.1D
W. O. Hassall, *They Saw it Happen 55BC-1485*, Blackwell, 1956: 6B
Nigel Kelly, *Medieval Realms*, Heinemann Educational, 1993: 8.1A
Geoffrey Keynes, *The Apologie and Treatise of Ambrose Paré*, Falcon
Educational Books, 1951: 9.3J, 9.3K, 9.3L, 9.3M
Hugh Lloyd Jones, *The Greek World*, Penguin, 1965: 5.6(1)
W.H.S. Jones, *Pliny's Natural History*, Heinemann, 1923: 5.6(2)
M. V. Lyons, *Medicine in the Medieval World*, Macmillan, 1984: 8.2B,
8.2C, 8.5K
R. H. Major, *Classic Descriptions of Disease*, Charles S. Thompson Inc.,
1945: 8.7P, 8.7S, 8.7V, 8.7W
V. Nutton, 'A Social History of Graeco-Roman Medicine', in *Medicine in
Society* (ed A. Wear) CUP, 1994: 5.2B
E.D. Phillips, *Greek Medicine*, Thames and Hudson, 1975: 4.2E, 4.5H,
4.5J, 4.5(1)
Colin Platt, *The English Medieval Town*, Granada, 1979: 8.6N
Dodie Poynter, *History at Source: Medicine 300-1929*, Evans Bros., 1971:
11.5(4)
Robert Reid, *Microbes and Men*, BBC, 1974: 11.6 (2 & 3), 12.2I
Philip Rhodes, *An Outline of the History of Medicine*, Butterworths,1985: 12.4
J. D. de C. M. Saunders & Charles D. O'Malley, *The Illustrations for the
Works of Andreas Vesalius*, World Publishing, 1950, 9.2D
SCHP, *Medicine Through Time: A Study in Development*, Book 1, Holmes
McDougal, 1976: 8.7P, 8.7Q, 8.7R
SCHP, *Medicine Through Time: A Study in Development*, Book 3, Holmes
McDougal, 1976: 811.4P, 13.1I
Joe Scott, *Medicine Through Time*, Holmes McDougal, 1987: 11.1G
Dr Thomas Shapter, *A History of the Cholera in Exeter in 1832*, 1841: 13.1D
Richard Shyrock, *The Development of Modern Medicine*, 1948: 12.6(2)
1962: 4.7M
Charles Singer, *Galen On Anatomical Procedures*, London 1956: 5.5K
G. Sweetman, *A History of Wincanton*, 1903: 11.1D
Hugh Thomas, *Spain*, 1964: 7.2A
Lynn Thorndike, *Michael Scot*, Nelson, 1965: 8.3E
R. Vallery-Radot, *Life of Pasteur*, London, 1911: 11.2H
J. J. Walsh, *Medieval Medicine*, 1920: 6C
Leo M. Zimmermann & Ilza Veith, *Great Ideas in the History of Surgery*,
1961: 12.2K

CONTENTS

CHAPTER 1

PREHISTORIC MEDICINE

1.1 What was the prehistoric period?

Look at the timeline below. It shows the time covered in this book. Most of the time is **prehistoric** (before people wrote things down). This makes it difficult for historians to know what happened.

The start of writing

History started as soon as people learnt to write. This happened at different times in different parts of the world. Writing started in Egypt long before it started in Britain. So Egypt had a written history when Britain was still prehistoric.

What makes people prehistoric?

- They were nomads (moved from place to place).
- They were hunter gatherers. They hunted animals and picked fruit and berries for food.
- They lived in small groups. There were no towns or roads.
- They had simple tools made from wood, bone or stone.
- They had no writing.

Over many thousands of years two things changed. One was farming. People grew food and stayed in one place. The other was making metal tools.

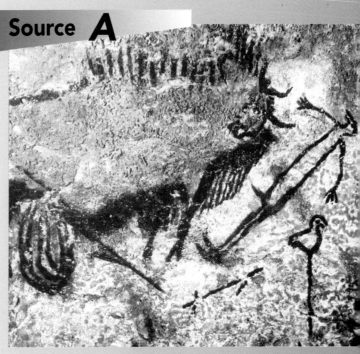

Source A

▲ A cave painting made by prehistoric people in France about 15,000 years ago.

CAVE PAINTINGS

Cave paintings are thought to show many different things. The human figure on the ground in front of the bison in Source A has been seen as a hunter, a human sacrifice and a shaman. We cannot know which of these is the one that the prehistoric artist meant to paint.

	Old Stone Age			New Stone Age		Bronze Age	Iron Age
8000 BC	15000 BC	12000 BC	9000 BC	6000 BC	3000 BC	0	AD 2000

Cave paintings in France
Sources A and C

▲ **The Stone Age (in most of Europe and the Middle East).**

1.2 Prehistoric medicine

We have found the bones of prehistoric peoples. These bones can show that people fell ill or were hurt. We do not know if they used medicine to get better.

Source B

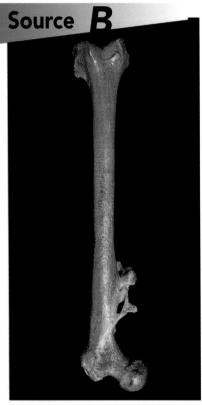

▲ The thigh bone of a prehistoric person. You can clearly see a large growth on the bone.

Source C

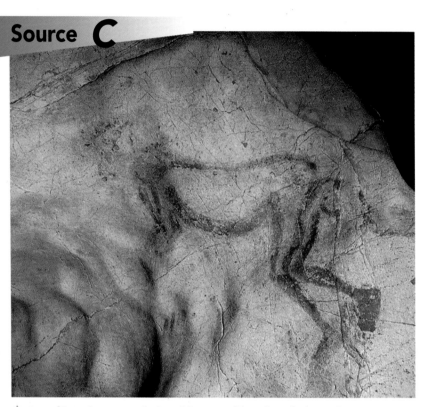

▲ A prehistoric cave painting. Many prehistoric paintings show a man with antlers like this one.

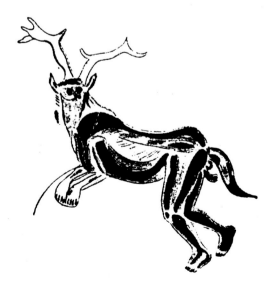

▶ This modern drawing of the cave painting in Source C shows the outline of a man with antlers, possibly wearing a mask, more clearly.

1.3 Trephined skulls: a prehistoric operation

Prehistoric graves of men and women have been found all over the world. The whole skeleton is in the grave. Sometimes there is evidence of trephining. This is when a hole is cut in a person's skull when they are still alive. Often the missing disc of bone is in the grave too. It may have a hole in it as if it had been worn as a lucky **charm**. Most trephined skulls have rounded edges around the holes. This shows that the person lived for some years after the operation. No children's skulls have been found with holes in them.

Why did prehistoric people cut holes in the heads of living men and women? Historians have puzzled over this for many years. There are four main theories (ideas).

The four main theories about trephining
Theory 1
Dr. Prunieres (1865) suggested the holes were made in the skulls so that they became drinking cups.
Theory 2
Professor Paul Broca (1876) suggested the trephining operation was done on children. Prehistoric people thought that those children who lived on had magical powers.
Theory 3
E. Guiard (1930) suggested trephining was to help illness, such as broken skulls, epilepsy and headaches.
Theory 4
Douglas Guthrie (1945) suggested trephining was to let out evil spirits.

PAUL BROCA

Paul Broca (1824–80) was a surgeon, anthropologist and archaeologist. He studied the brain.

In medicine, he discovered parts of the brain which, when damaged, made it hard for people to understand and explain ideas. He also found the part of the brain that controls a person's ability to talk. This part of the brain was named after him.

Broca was interested in prehistoric peoples' brains. He measured many modern and prehistoric skulls. He worked out the size and shape of the brains of different prehistoric peoples. Different parts of the brain control different skills. So, Broca said, you should be able to work out what skills prehistoric people had from the size and shape of their brains.

Source D

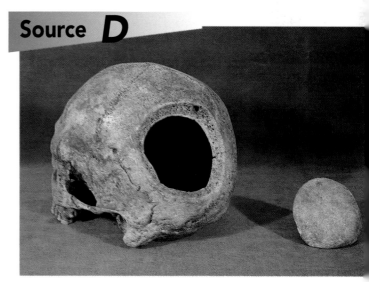

▲ A prehistoric skull. The hole was cut out while the person was alive. We know this because the bone grew afterwards – rounding off the edge.

What do we know about prehistoric medicine?

We know there was some illness. We know that trephining operations were done. But we do not know what prehistoric people thought about illness and medicine. One way to find out is to look at people who have lived in prehistoric ways until recently. This is not the whole answer but it may help.

The Aborigines of Australia

Until about 100 years ago, the Aborigines lived in a way that was in many ways prehistoric. They had no form of writing. They were nomads. They hunted and gathered their food.

Causes of illness – obvious and spirit

The Aborigines felt that some things had an obvious cause. If a person fell and broke her arm it was covered in clay. The clay then set hard so the bone could heal. But some illnesses did not have an obvious cause. The Aborigines believed that such illnesses were caused by spirits.

Aboriginal spirits

The Aborigines thought the world started in the **dreamtime**. This was when the spirit ancestors lived. These spirits controlled many things. They controlled new life. They controlled where a stream flowed. If a person was sick for no obvious reason, then maybe the sickness was controlled by a spirit.

Spirit causes of illness

The Aborigines had two spirit explanations for sickness. The first was that an evil spirit had entered the sick person's body. The second was that the sick person's spirit had left the body.

If an evil spirit had entered a sick person, the evil spirit had to be driven out. If an enemy had taken the sick person's spirit (possibly using a special bone) the treatment was to find the bone which would have the sick person's spirit stuck to it. Only a spirit treatment would cure a spirit illness.

THE PREHISTORIC PERIOD

Historians divide the prehistoric period into:

Old Stone Age [Palaeolithic] when people were nomadic hunter-gatherers.

New Stone Age [Neolithic] when farming and living in one place became common.

Bronze Age when metal tools were first used.

Iron Age when iron improved the tools and weapons which could be made.

There was an overlap in time between the prehistoric period and those described in the next chapters. For instance, Britain was in the Iron Age during the Greek and early Roman periods.

Source **E**

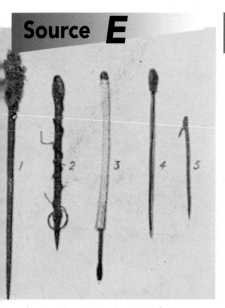

▲ A collection of pointing bones and sticks. When tipped with gum and used in ceremonies they were said to control spirits.

Source **F**

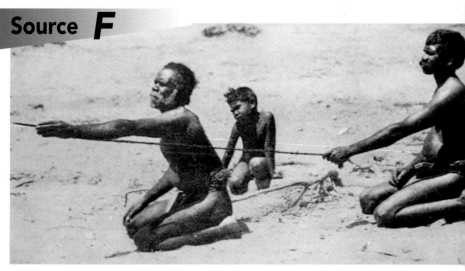

▲ Aborigines using a death bone. This was said to send spirits to kill over long distances.

EARLY ARCHAEOLOGISTS

Western scholars used to believe that the world had been created in 4004 BC, a date worked out from the Bible. But by the 19th century, people were starting to make sense of the evidence before their eyes. We now call this knowledge the sciences of geology and archaeology.

First Charles Lyell wrote of the geological signs that the Earth was ancient. His book came out in the 1830s. Then Charles Darwin showed that, instead of being created in one day, animals had evolved over time . His important book *The Origin of Species* was published in 1859.

Archaeologists studying cave dwellings in France and England showed that mankind was much older than 4004 BC.

Our present view of prehistory as a very long period with slow developments was first suggested in 1865 by John Lubbock in his book *Pre-historic Times*.

1.5 Conclusions

We know a little about the way prehistoric people lived. We know this from finding their tools, graves and skeletons. The Aborigines lived in a similar way. So, maybe we can learn about prehistoric medicine from looking at the medicine of the Aborigines.

Obvious and spirit reasons for illness

The Aborigines looked at illness in two ways. So maybe the prehistoric people looked at illness in two ways. Maybe they believed that some illnesses were caused by spirits. Maybe trephining was a way to let an evil spirit out of a sick person's head. But we can never really know what people thought, because there are no written records,

In 1915–16 and 1917–8, Bronislaw Malinowski lived among the Trobriand Islanders near New Guinea in Melanesia. He lived in a tent, spoke the islanders' language, and recorded their lives and belief systems. Malinowski describes human beings who make sense of their environment with limited scientific and technical information. Prehistoric communities may well have held similar ideas.

The Islanders lived in small villages. Their economy was based on pigs, fishing, and yams. Each village centred on the chief's house and a store house for yams. Magic played a very important part in the Islanders' lives as these extracts from Malinowski's writings show.

Health to the Melanesians is a natural state of affairs, and they believe that, unless tampered with, the human body will remain in perfect order. But they know there are natural means which can affect health and even destroy the body. Poisons, wounds, burns, falls are known to cause disablement or death in a natural way. They believe there are different ways to the nether world for those who died by sorcery and those who met 'natural' death.

Again, it is recognized that cold, heat, overstrain, too much sun, overeating, can all cause minor ailments, which are treated by natural remedies such as massage, steaming, warming at a fire and certain potions.

By far the most causes of illness and death are ascribed to sorcery. The line of distinction between sorcery and the other causes is clear in theory and in most cases of practice, but it must be realized that it is subject to what could be called the personal perspective. That is, the more closely a case has to do with the person who considers it, the less will it be 'natural,' the more 'magical.' Thus a very old man, whose pending death will be considered natural by the other members of the community, will be afraid only of sorcery and never think of his natural fate. A fairly sick person will diagnose sorcery in his own case, while all the others might speak of too much betel nut or overeating or some other indulgence.

[Bronislaw Malinowski, *Magic, Science and Religion*, 1948.]

Source 1

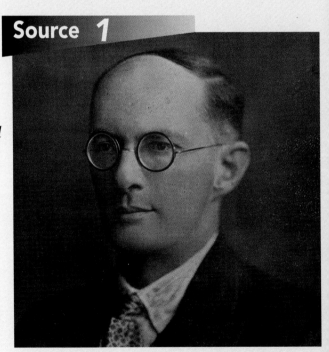

▲ **Bronislaw Malinowski**

CHAPTER 2

EGYPTIAN MEDICINE

2.1 Ancient Egypt

Life in Ancient Egypt
3000BC–400BC
Life in Egypt was well organized.

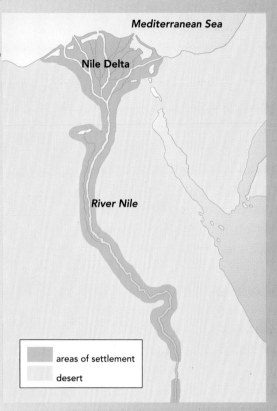

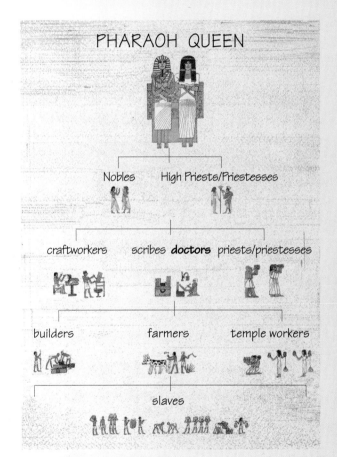

Prehistoric people did not write. Egyptian people did write. Egyptian doctors could write down any cures they discovered. Then other doctors could learn from the first doctor.

Egyptian religion
The Egyptians believed their gods did everything. From making the sun rise to causing and curing illness.

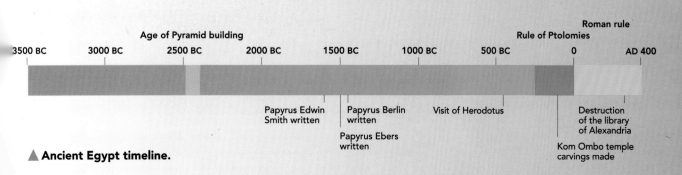

▲ Ancient Egypt timeline.

Causes of disease

Like prehistoric people, the Egyptians thought that many diseases were caused by evil spirits entering the body. They often wore **charms** to keep evil spirits away.

Medical books

The Egyptians wrote books so we know what they thought about disease. The earliest medical books have been lost. But we do have many later ones. Some of the books are only lists of magical spells for getting rid of evil spirits. Some books, though, tell us about operations, medicines, hygiene and diets for sick people.

Medicine and spells

Egyptians made medicines from minerals, animals and plants such as coriander, garlic and figs. The medicines were cooked up and mixed with wine, beer or water (sometimes sweetened with honey). Chest diseases were treated by making the patient breathe in steam. Cuts were covered with ointment.

The doctor often gave medicine and said a **spell**. Together the medicine and spell drove the evil spirits away from the sick person. The doctor did exactly what the medical books said. If the doctor did not do this and the patient died, the doctor might be killed.

The medical books show that, if a cure worked, the doctors kept using it.

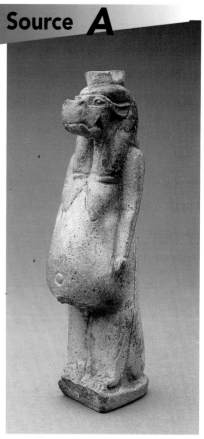

Source A

▲ A charm or amulet of the goddess of childbirth. She was called Tawaret. Her face is fierce to drive away evil spirits which hurt the mother or baby.

▶ A spell from the *Papyrus Ebers*, a medical book, written about 1500 BC. The doctor chanted the spell while giving the medicine.

Source B

Here is the great remedy. Come! You who drive evil things out. He who drinks this shall be cured.

THOTH

Egyptians first saw Thoth as the moon god who looked after the goddess Osiris when she was pregnant, and healed her son, Horus. Later, he was worshipped as the god of learning. Egyptians said Thoth invented writing and language. He is often shown with a human body and the head of an ibis.

EGYPTIAN MEDICAL BOOKS

The Ancient Egyptians wrote on papyrus [a kind of paper made from reeds]. A few medical books have survived from that time. They are called after the owner or the museum where they are kept.

The *Papyrus Ebers*, written about 1500 BC is called after a German, Maurice Ebers.

The *Papyrus Edwin Smith* was bought by Smith in 1862. It was written in about 1600 BC. The books contain, spells, medicines, and advice on surgery.

2.3 Religion and anatomy

Anatomy and religion

The Egyptians found out how bodies were made (**anatomy**) because they had to cut up bodies as part of their religion. They believed that when a person died the soul left the body for a while. Then the soul came back and the person began an afterlife. So it was very important to preserve the dead body so that the soul could get back in.

Source C

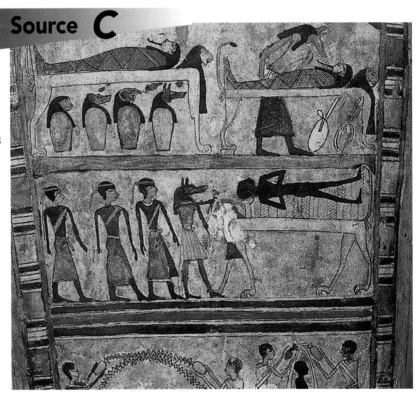

▲ A painted coffin dated about 600 BC. At the bottom the body is being washed in a natron (salt) solution. In the middle the body is covered with natron crystals during the 40 day drying-out stage. At the top, on the left, the embalmed body (called a mummy) is in the tomb above four jars. The jars hold the liver, lungs, stomach and intestines. On the right the god, Anubis, is with the mummy.

Source D

Forty-six vessels go from the heart to every limb. Wherever a doctor places his hands he hears the heart.

▲ From the *Papyrus Ebers*, about 1500 BC.

Embalming but not dissecting

The Egyptians preserved dead bodies by soaking them in different liquids, covering them in oils and wrapping them in bandages. This was called **embalming**.

The Egyptians understood a great deal about bodies because they cut them open to embalm them. They knew where organs like the heart and lungs were.

But they did not do any more cutting up. This was because they believed that the body must be kept for a life after death.

2.4 A natural theory of the causes of disease

A new, natural theory

The River Nile was vital to life in Egypt. Without the river and its seasoned flooding, no crops could be grown.

The Egyptians looked at the River Nile with all its channels and ditches. Perhaps the human body was like this. Perhaps it was full of channels and ditches carrying blood and food and water around it. If these channels got blocked a person would become ill. Doctors, who believed in this idea, used a number of treatments.

To clear the blocks

- Some doctors thought that making the patient sick would clear the blockage.
- Purges (**laxatives**) were use to clear the lower end of the body.
- Bleeding was also used. The doctor cut open a vein to clear the blood channels.

Natural and spiritual causes of disease side by side

Not all doctors liked the idea of channels in the body. Some kept to the idea of spirits causing disease.

The *Papyrus Ebers*, a medical book, gives spells for getting rid of illness.

It also lists herbs to use to get sick people better. Often the herbs helped to unblock the channels.

Source F

If he is ill in his arm then make him vomit. Bandage his fingers with water melon. If he is ill in the bowel the blockage must be cleared. Colocynth, senna and fruit of sycamore are made into a paste for him to eat.

▲ Treatment from the *Papyrus Ebers*, about 1500 BC.

2.5 Surgery

Surgery

Doctors passed their jobs on from father to son (or sometimes daughter). Some doctors may have carried out small surgical operations but probably not major ones.

Minor operations

The *Papyrus Edwin Smith* described some of these simple operations. The Egyptians set dislocated arms and legs. They set broken bones. They cut away small cysts and tumours. They used the leaves and bark of the willow tree to bind up wounds. We now know that willow is a kind of **antiseptic**. It helped to stop wounds going bad. This meant that many people probably recovered from these small operations.

Source G

If a man has a dislocation of the jaw and cannot close it, put your thumbs on the ends of the two rami of the lower jawbone, inside the mouth. Put your fingers under his chin and make them fall back into the correct position.

▲ From the *Papyrus Edwin Smith*, about 1600 BC.

Source H

When you come across a swelling that moves under your moving finger and the patient is clammy, then you say, 'I will treat with fire since cautery heals it.'

When a swelling is like a hard stone under your fingers, then you say, 'I will treat the disease with a knife.'

▲ From the *Papyrus Ebers*, about 1500 BC.

Source I

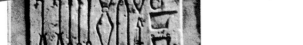

◀ A carving showing Egyptian surgical instruments. These include saws, forceps, scalpels and scissors. They were usually made from bronze, although some surgical knives were made of flint.

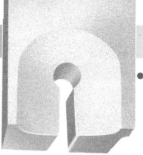

▲ An artist's reconstruction of an Egyptian toilet seat made of limestone.

Keeping clean

The Egyptians washed every day. The priests washed even more often. Maybe keeping clean had more to do with religion than with health. But, whatever the reason, keeping clean helped the Egyptians to keep healthy.

Water

The Egyptians used the water from the River Nile to water their crops. They had lots of ditches carrying the river water to the fields. But they did not have water flushed toilets. Toilets were a stone seat over a jar. Rich people had baths but these just drained into a jar too. The jars could be taken to the fields by slaves. This manured and watered the fields.

Source J

The Egyptians drink from cups of bronze which they clean daily. They keep their clothes clean.

Their priests shave their whole bodies and wash three times a day.

▲ From *The Histories* by the Greek historian Herodotus, about 450 BC.

HERODOTUS

Herodotus (c484–c425 BC) was born in modern Turkey, then part of the Greek world. He later lived in Athens and travelled all over the Mediterranean. He eventually settled in Thurii, a Greek colony in Italy. He lived there until he died.

Herodotus is the first great historian of the ancient world. *The Histories* tells the story of the Greek and Persian wars. In this book Herodotus tries to look at accounts critically and find out the truth.

His writings on Egypt are from notes he used to write *The Histories*. At first he wanted to write a book about the geography of the Mediterranean world, but he changed his mind.

We do not know exactly when Herodotus visited Egypt. From what he says in the book we know that he was there from August to December. He talks about seeing unburied skulls on the battlefield at Papremis. This means he must have gone there after the battle, which took place in 460 BC.

When the book became a history series, the notes on Egypt took up a whole book. They did not really fit in with his history, but Herodotus used them anyway.

Herodotus wrote his book for people who had never been to Egypt, so he described everything in great detail. That makes it very useful for historians today.

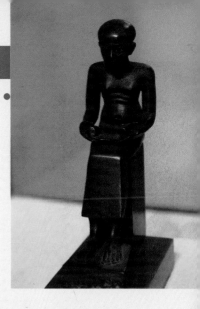

Imhotep lived and worked about 2600 BC. He was the vizier (chief minister) of King Zoser, a pharaoh of the Third Dynasty. He was in overall charge of running the country. This is the same position as Joseph holds in the Bible story. Imhotep was not just an administrator. He was also an astronomer, architect, author, priest and doctor.

Imhotep is thought to have been responsible for building the Step Pyramid at Saqqara, the first great stone building in Egypt. This was where King Zoser was buried. It was the centre of an elaborate complex of monuments. The complex was surrounded by a 10m high stone wall, 544m by 277m. Inside, as well as the pyramid, was a courtyard, temples, chapels, and smaller buildings. The word pyramid comes to us from the Greeks. They used their word *pyramis*, meaning wheat cakes, to describe the buildings – they were a similar shape. The Egyptian word for pyramid was *mer*, which could be translated as 'place of ascension'. The step pyramid may have been intended to represent a staircase from which Zoser could ascend to the heavens, and down which he could return to live his life after death.

Imhotep's tomb became a temple of healing. It is also now lost, and a major archaeological expedition to find it in 1965 found instead the buried complexes of the sacred ibises, falcons, baboons, and cows which played an important part in Egyptian religion.

The worship of Imhotep continued throughout the Egyptian period. If anything he became a more important god from about 500 BC onwards. Many statues of him have been found, usually showing him reading a scroll. There were major temples dedicated to his worship at Memphis, Thebes and Philæ.

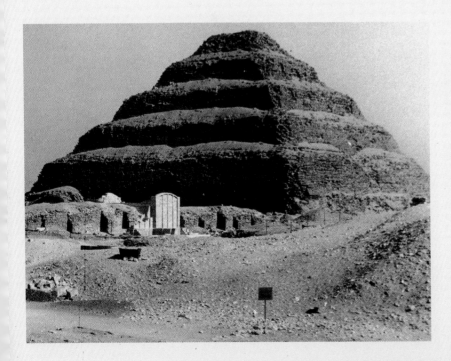

CHAPTER 3

MINOAN CRETE

3.1 Who were the Minoans?

The Minoans lived on the island of Crete. Their civilization was at its best about 3,000 years ago.

Archaeologists have found many Minoan buildings.

We also know about the Minoans from Greek writers.

Minoan hygiene

Archaeologists have found several Minoan palaces. The most famous is at Knossos.

They have found water tanks to collect rain water. They have also found lavatories and drains, which took away the sewage.

▼**One of the stone drains at the Minoan palace of Knossos. It carried dirty water away.**

Source A

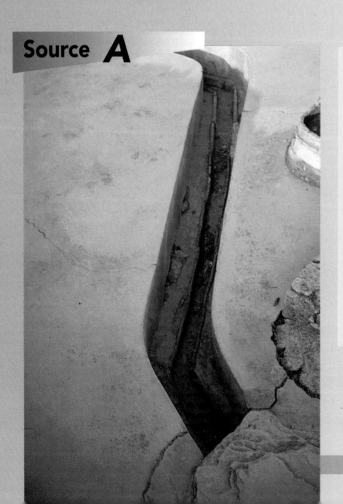

SIR ARTHUR EVANS

The Minoan palace of Knossos was excavated by Sir Arthur Evans.

Evans bought land in Crete. In 1900, he began digging and found the large palace at Knossos.

He found room after room. He worked out what he thought the rooms were used for.

Archaeologists today do not agree with all of his ideas.

Aqueducts?

Some of the pipes at Knossos might have brought water from far away. It is possible that the Minoans built **aqueducts** (bridges which carry water) to cross valleys. No one knows for certain.

3.2 The legacy of the Minoans

The Minoan palaces destroyed

The palaces were destroyed by fire over 3,000 years ago.

No one knows what destroyed them. Some historians think a volcano erupted nearby and set off earthquakes. Others think that the Greeks attacked and burnt the palaces.

What happened to the Minoans?

No one knows. But all the skill of the Minoans in building water systems was lost. No one built water systems and aqueducts until Roman times. This loss of knowledge is called regression. Knowledge lost had to be rediscovered later.

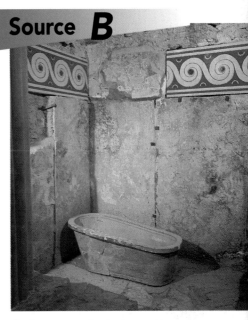

Source **B**

▲ **The Queen's bathroom at Knossos.**

CHANCE

Many changes happen by **chance**. This means that they happen by accident, not because someone has set out to make them happen.

If the Minoan civilization had not been destroyed then their ideas about keeping clean could have been passed on.

The progress of medicine was held up by the collapse of the Minoan civilization. No one intended this to happen.

KING MINOS

The Minoans are named after King Minos. Greek myths say Minos was the son of the god Zeus who ruled Crete. The myths say that Minos kept a Minotaur (a creature that was half man, half bull) in a maze of passages under his palace. The drainage system under the Palace of Knossos looks very like a maze.

CHAPTER 4

ANCIENT GREECE

4.1 Greece 1000 BC – 300 BC

Ancient Greece was not one country. The Greek people lived on the land and islands around the eastern Mediterranean (see map). They built many cities. Each city ruled itself. Sometimes they fought each other.

Greek language and gods

Greek people spoke the same language, wherever they lived. They believed in the same gods. The gods were a way of explaining how the world worked.

Why there was winter

Demeter was the goddess of agriculture. Her daughter had to spend half the year in the underworld. This made Demeter angry. She did not allow plants to grow while her daughter was in the underworld. So this made the winter time.

Why there were volcanoes

The god of fire was a blacksmith. His name was Hephaestos. He made the smoke and fire of volcanoes. This was when he was working at his forge.

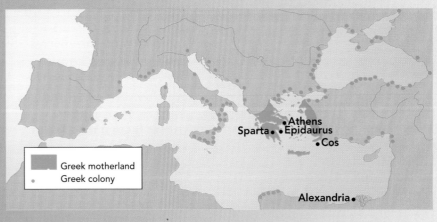

◀ **The Greek world, in about 450 BC. Alexandria is in Egypt at the mouth of the River Nile.**

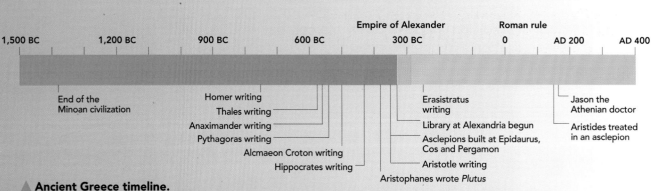

▲ **Ancient Greece timeline.**

Greek civilization 600 BC – 300 BC

Greek people were rich and powerful at this time. They made money from trade and farming. Some people were very rich. They did not have to work. So they had plenty of time to enjoy themselves. They also had plenty of time to think.

Pythagoras and other great thinkers

Pythagoras had completely new ideas in mathematics. He thought up a new theorem. Thales of Miletus studied astronomy and put forward the idea that water was the basis of life. Anaximander used this idea about water to work out his own ideas. He said all things were made from four **elements** – water, fire, earth and air.

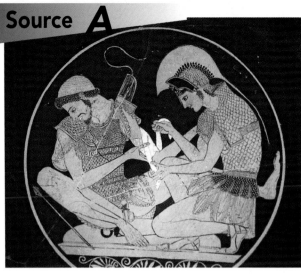

▲ **A hero from the siege of Troy treats his wounded friend. This painting is from a decorated cup.**

CHANGE AND DEVELOPMENT

A **change** is a completely new idea.

A **development** is when something is based on what went before it – it has *developed* from a previous idea.

Greek medicine

We first know about Greek medicine from the poems of Homer. He wrote about war and treating wounded soldiers. Later, more Greek people wrote about medicine. One of the most famous was **Hippocrates**.

Rational medicine and supernatural medicine

Hippocrates was interested in **rational** medicine. He wanted to work out why things happened. He wrote a number of books about medicine in about 430 BC.

The other sort of medicine was **supernatural** medicine. This was to do with spirits and the god Asclepios. This kind of medicine was very popular around and after 400 BC.

ANAXIMANDER

Anaximander was born in 610 BC, in Militus, part of the Greek world. He studied astronomy and drew the first map of the known world.

He said that everything, from plants to the air, from stones to people, was made from the same thing. This was called *apeiron*. He said that apeiron slowly separated into the four elements: earth, air, fire and water. His ideas about people having the four elements in them was built into the theory of the four humours.

Supernatural medicine

Asclepios was the Greek god of healing. The Greeks built temples to worship him. Sick people would go to one of the temples. They spent at least one night there. The sick person would probably have:

- Given a gift to the god Asclepios.
- Washed in the sea.
- Slept in a part of the temple called the *abaton*.

The sick person expected to be visited by Asclepios. Some people had dreams. Probably the priests treated people while they were asleep. The snake was Asclepios' sacred animal. Sometimes the priests used snakes as part of the treatment.

How we know

Sick people were supposed to wake up cured. Sometimes they did. Sometimes they did not. Aristides, who came from Athens, visited many temples of Asclepios. He wrote about some treatment he had in AD 150. Aristophanes also wrote about treatment in a play called *Plutus* in about 370 BC.

Source B

First we had to bathe Plutus in the sea.

Then we entered the temple and gave our offerings. There were many sick people. Soon the temple priest put out the light and told us to sleep. The god sat down by Plutus. He wiped his head and eyelids.

Next Panacea [the god's daughter] covered his face with a scarlet cloth. The god whistled and two snakes came.

They licked Plutus' eyelids and he could see again. But the god and his helpers had gone.

▲ From *Plutus*, a play written by Aristophanes. Plutus was cured of blindness.

Source C

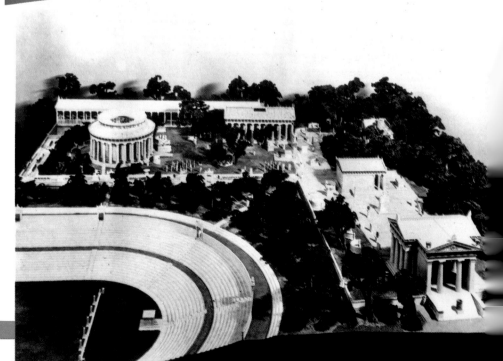

▶ A model of the temple to Asclepios at Epidaurus.

Continuity

For hundreds of years sick people visited religious places. They wanted to be cured. Sick people visited the temples of Asclepios from about 300 BC to about AD 400. In the Middle Ages, in Britain and Europe, sick people visited great churches. Until a few years ago sick people in parts of Greece, Italy and Sicily spent the night in a church. They all hoped to be cured.

We are looking at **change** in the history of medicine. But it is important to know that there was **continuity** too.

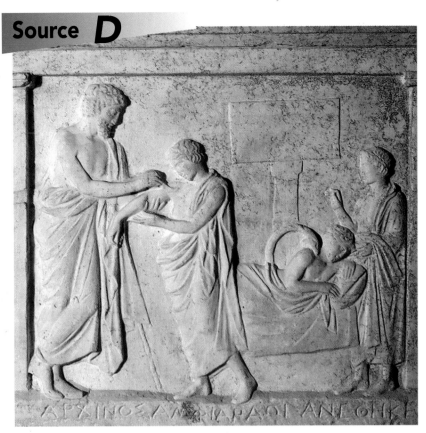

▲ A carving showing Asclepios treating a boy called Archinos. This was made about 350 BC.

Source **E**

- Ambrosia became blind in one eye. She had laughed at cures before. But she dreamed Asclepios said he would cure her if she gave a silver pig. He seemed to cut into her eyeball and pour in medicine. When she woke she was cured.

- Euhippus had a spear point in his jaw for six years. As he was sleeping in the temple Asclepios pulled it out.

- While a man slept in the temple a snake licked his diseased toe. He woke cured.

▲ Writings in stone, called *Iamata*, at a temple to Asclepios. Many such writings recording cures have been found.

ARISTOPHANES

Aristophanes (c 450 BC – c 388 BC) was a famous Greek playwright.

Aristophanes wrote more than 40 plays. He lived in Athens. His plays make fun of the political goings-on in that city. They also make fun of some of the sorts of people who lived there.

Plutus is about a poor man who helps a blind man. The blind man is the god of wealth in disguise. When he has been cured he rewards the poor man for his help.

Hippocrates and balance

Hippocrates learnt from two earlier thinkers called Pythagoras and Alcmaeon of Croton. They taught that a body was healthy when all the parts were in balance, and neither too hot nor too cold.

The Hippocratic Corpus (books)

Hippocrates left a collection of medical books called the *Hippocratic Corpus*. He probably did not write all of them himself. The books are important because they tell us about Greek medicine.

What Hippocrates did not want

Hippocrates did not want doctors to think that illness was caused or cured by magic. He also did not want doctors to have just one theory about illness which fitted every patient.

What Hippocrates did want

Hippocrates wanted doctors to watch their sick patients carefully and to treat them according to what was going on. This is called **clinical observation**. This was not a new idea. The Egyptians had also believed in watching the patient for symptoms. For instance, doctors should watch a patient with a cold. Then next time they would know what was likely to happen and what to do about it.

CLINICAL OBSERVATION

A doctor watches all the changes in a person during an illness.

Diagnosis
What's wrong? (sneezing)

Prognosis
What is going to happen? (after sneezing comes shivering)

Observation
Keep watching. (after shivering comes coughing)

Treatment
The doctor should give medicine only when he is sure of what is wrong with the sick person.

▶ The tombstone of Jason, a doctor from Athens, who died in the 2nd century AD. Jason is shown examining a patient.

Source **F**

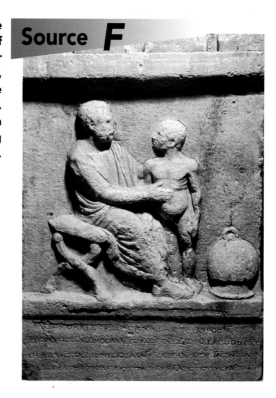

Hippocrates also said sick people should be kept clean and quiet. A doctor should only give medicine if he was sure he knew what was wrong with the patient.

Surgery

The Greeks did not allow anyone to cut up dead bodies. So surgeons did not know where things were inside the body. This was dangerous for the patient! Most surgery was simple, such as setting breaks and resetting dislocated bones.

Source G

A person with quinsey shivers, has a headache, swelling under the jaw and dry mouth.

He cannot spit or breathe lying down. He must be bled and made to breathe in a mixture of vinegar and soda heated in oil and water. Hot sponges must be put on his neck.

He must gargle herbs and have his throat cleaned out.

▲ From a Hippocratic book called *On Diseases*.

4.4 The four humours

Aristotle (384–322 BC)

Many Hippocratic books said that bodies needed to be in balance to be well. Some of the books talked about balancing **four humours**. However, Aristotle took the ideas much further.

He said that the body was made up of four liquids or humours. Each humour was connected to a season (see diagram).

The body could get out of balance. For instance, lots of people got colds in winter. They had too much phlegm.

The right treatment by the doctor was to give medicines to clear the phlegm.

This would bring the four humours back into balance in the body.

A person with a hot fever probably had too much blood in the body. In this case the doctor would cut a vein and take some blood out of the body. This was called 'bleeding' the patient.

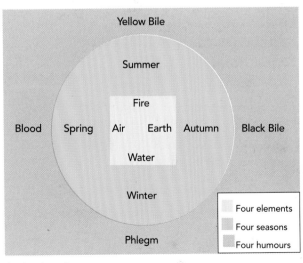

▲ The four humours.

Alexander the Great

Alexander the Great conquered a lot of land. He built a great, new city in Egypt in 332 BC. He called it **Alexandria**. The city became famous for its library. It also became a great place for the study of medicine. Many doctors were trained at Alexandria.

The study of medicine – dissection

The Greeks did not allow dissection of dead bodies. But thinkers like Aristotle said that the soul of a dead person left the body. It did not matter if you cut up the dead body.

Dissection in Alexandria

Not everyone liked Aristotle's ideas. However, dissection was allowed in Alexandria. Doctors learned a lot about bodies. For a time even live bodies were cut up. These were criminals who were going to be executed. In this way the doctors saw how the blood moved in the veins.

Was surgery safer?

Doctors in Alexandria knew a lot more about bodies. However, having an operation was still very dangerous. There were no **anaesthetics** and no one knew much about keeping wounds clean.

New ideas

Herophilus (about 335 BC–280 BC) put forward the idea that the nerves were channels that carried the life force or **pneuma**.

Erasistratus (about 250 BC) studied the human body and noted the difference between arteries, veins and nerves. He found that the nerves were solid so he said that they could not carry pneuma.

Source *H*

Chest trouble starts with sweating, a salty, bitter mouth, pains in the ribs and shoulder blades, shaking hands and dry cough. Treat with pounded radishes, cardamons, mustard, purslane and rocket in warm water. This will cause a healing vomit.

▲ From a book by Diocles, a Greek doctor who lived in Alexandria in the 4th century BC.

HEROPHILUS

Herophilus (c 335 BC – c 280 BC) worked in Alexandria when human dissection was allowed. He studied the human brain. He also studied the eyes and the digestive system.

Herophilus believed in the idea of keeping the body healthy by keeping it in balance. He stressed the value of taking exercise and eating the right sorts of food. He also thought that herbal cures and drugs should be used to help to keep the body in balance.

His writings were destroyed when the library at Alexandria burned down. His ideas were passed on by others like Galen.

Source I

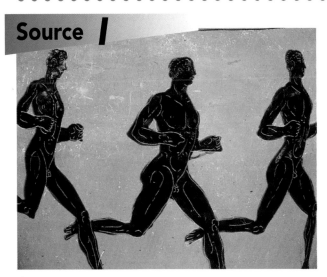

▲ A vase painting, from 333 BC. It shows young men racing. The Greeks thought that exercise kept people healthy.

Keeping healthy

The Greeks said that eating and drinking affected your health. Exercise, work and sleep affected your health.

Hippocratic books

Some of the books set out what a person should eat or not eat. How much a person drank was important. They said how much exercise a person should take. They said keeping clean was important. So was getting enough sleep.

Many doctors told their patients how to live a healthy life. This was better than waiting until they were ill and then taking medicine.

Source J

After waking, a man should wait a little. Then get up. He should rub his body with oil. Then wash in pure water.

He should rub his teeth with his finger using peppermint powder. He should oil his nose, ears and hair every day. And wash his hair less often.

After this he should go to work. If he does not need to work, he should go for a walk. This clears out the body. He is then ready to eat.

▲ From a book by Diocles, a Greek doctor.

Source K

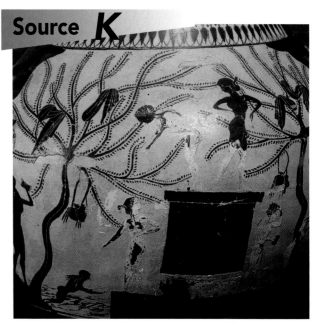

► A vase painting, from about 450 BC. It shows women washing.

The spread of Greek medicine

Greek doctors travelled all around the lands by the Mediterranean Sea. Other doctors learnt from the Greeks. Over the years Greek ideas about medicine spread far and wide.

A code of conduct – the Hippocratic Oath

Hippocrates said it was very important that a doctor behaved well. He should take an **oath** to do his best.

The idea that doctors should behave well is still followed today.

Clinical observation

The Greeks said that clinical observation was very important. Doctors should always see a patient before giving medicine. Records should be kept of a patient's illnesses.

All these things are still done today.

Source L

▲ A Greek painted vase, from about 400 BC. The doctor is sitting in the centre of the painting. To his right is a man he is about to bleed. There is a large bowl on the floor to catch the blood.

Source M

I swear by Apollo, by Asclepios, and by all the gods and goddesses that I will carry out this oath.

I will use treatment to help the sick according to my ability and judgment but never with a view to injury or wrong-doing.

▲ A small part of the Hippocratic Oath quoted in D. Guthrie, *A History of Medicine*, 1945.

DIOCLES

Diocles worked as a doctor in the 4th century BC. He worked in Athens for most of his life. He was interested in anatomy but, because he lived in Athens, he could only dissect animals, not people.

Diocles wrote about diet and herbal cures. He also wrote books about the way the body worked. He had certainly read the Hippocratic books. He may even have been one of the people who helped to set up the collection (see page 24).

Diocles' books do not set out any new ideas about medicine. But they do set out new treatments. They are especially useful for the herbal cures they suggest.

Among the Hippocratic collection is the famous Hippocratic Oath. It outlines the proper way for doctors to behave. It was taken by all doctors in the western world as a matter of course until the first half of the 20th century. Some students still swear a version of it today.

There have been many different versions of the oath used over the centuries, but the guiding principles of ethical and discreet conduct have remained the same. From a historian's perspective it is interesting to see that even at this early age the oath suggests that surgeons and doctors had developed into two separate groups, and that doctors thought they should not do surgeon's work, probably because they thought it was beneath them.

Hippocratic Oath

I swear by Apollo the Physician, by Asclepios, by Hygeia, by Panacea, and by all the gods and goddesses that I will carry out this oath according to my ability and judgement.

The treatment I adopt shall be for the benefit of my patients according to my ability and judgement, and not for their hurt or for any wrong. I will give no deadly drug to any, though it be asked of me, nor will I counsel such, and I will not aid a woman to procure abortion. I will not use the knife, even upon sufferers of the stone, but I will give place to those that are craftsmen therein. Whatsoever house I enter, there will I go for the benefit of the sick, refraining from all wrongdoing or corruption, and especially from any act of seduction, of male or female, slave or free. Whatsoever things I shall see or hear concerning the life of men in my attendance on the sick or privately, which ought not to be noised abroad, I will keep silence thereon, counting such things to be as sacred secrets.

If I carry out this oath and break it not, may I gain forever reputation among all men for my life and for my art, but if I break it and forswear myself, may my lot be otherwise.

CHAPTER 5

ROMAN MEDICINE

5.1 Roman civilization

How Rome ruled

Rome conquered the rest of Italy. The Romans then conquered more and more land, and built up a huge **empire** (see map below). The Romans were well organized. They built good roads and used them to send officials and armies to govern their empire.

Usually everyone did what the government in Rome said because they were backed up by a large army. So it was important to keep the soldiers in this army healthy. The Romans thought a lot about how to prevent disease.

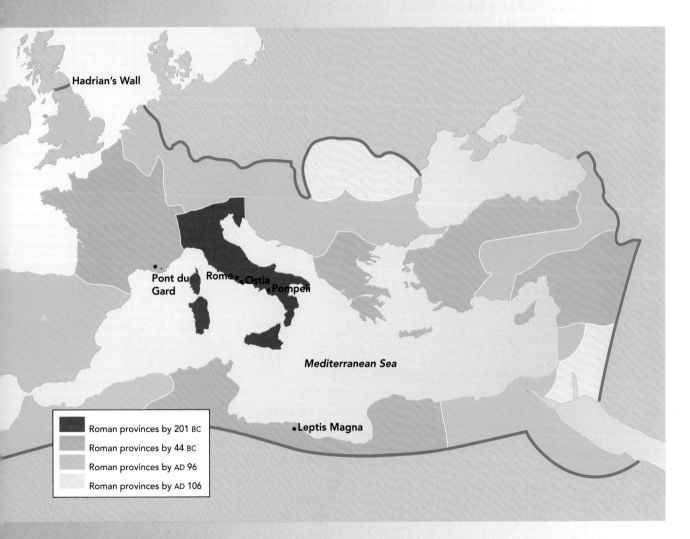

Hadrian's Wall

Pont du Gard

Rome

Ostia

Pompeii

Mediterranean Sea

Leptis Magna

Roman provinces by 201 BC
Roman provinces by 44 BC
Roman provinces by AD 96
Roman provinces by AD 106

▲ **The Roman Empire.**

5.2 Medicine in early Rome

Respect for doctors?

At first there were not many doctors in Rome. People treated their families with herbs, common sense (rest if you are ill) and some superstitious ideas. When Rome conquered Greece (about 250 BC) they took some Greeks back to Rome with them as slaves. Some of these were doctors. They only had a low status, but, gradually, more and more Romans went to see Greek doctors. They also used some Greek ideas on spiritual cures. They built a temple to Asclepios. This temple in Rome treated poor people and slaves.

Keeping people healthy

The Romans ruled many countries. They needed a big army to keep order. They needed the soldiers to be healthy. They set up hospitals for soldiers all over the Roman Empire. They also set up hospitals for the civil servants who collected taxes and kept the law. They paid state doctors to care for the poor.

Source A

They have sworn to kill all barbarians with their drugs, and they call us barbarians. I forbid you to use doctors.

▲ The Roman writer Cato, who died in 149 BC, warning his son against Greek doctors.

CATO

Marcus Porcius Cato (234 BC – 149 BC) was a Roman politician. He also wrote books.

Cato was worried about the rapid growth of the Roman Empire. He felt that Roman ways were being affected by new ideas from the lands they took over.

Cato was especially worried about Greek ideas. He thought that they were too popular. They were making the Romans less Roman. He thought that Romans should stick to the old ways.

Source B

Social and ethnic status of Roman doctors from the 1st to the 3rd century AD

	Total	Greek
Citizens	186	118
Freedmen (ex slaves)	170	158
Slaves	55	54
Foreign, non-citizens	31	23
Total	442	353

◄ This table lists all the doctors for whom tombstones have been found. Obviously this is not all the doctors for those 300 years. Based on figures in V. Nutton, *A Social History of Graeco-Roman Medicine*.

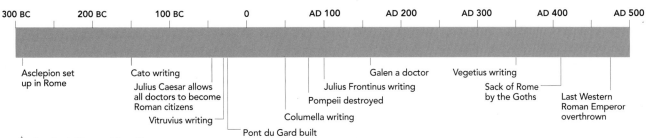

▲ Ancient Rome timeline.

300 BC | 200 BC | 100 BC | 0 | AD 100 | AD 200 | AD 300 | AD 400 | AD 500

Asclepion set up in Rome

Cato writing

Julius Caesar allows all doctors to become Roman citizens

Vitruvius writing

Pont du Gard built

Columella writing

Pompeii destroyed

Julius Frontinus writing

Galen a doctor

Vegetius writing

Sack of Rome by the Goths

Last Western Roman Emperor overthrown

Greek doctors become Roman citizens

Greek doctors still had low status, even if they were used more and more. Then, in 46 BC, Julius Caesar made a law that Greek doctors could become Roman citizens. Some Greek doctors became rich and famous.

5.3 Public health

How to keep healthy

The Romans noticed that people who lived near the marshes around Rome often died from a fever. We now call this fever, malaria. They built a temple to the goddess of fever and drained the marshes. Far fewer people got malaria.

What does this say about Roman public health?

1 The Romans did not know that mosquitoes who live in marshes spread malaria by biting human beings. However, the Romans saw that marshes were unhealthy so they got rid of them.

2 Draining the marshes was not easy or cheap. But the Romans were very clever, rich and well organized. They could take on large engineering work like draining marshes or building bridges.

Roman ideas about bad health

The Romans believed you could be made ill by:

- bad smells
- bad water
- marshes
- being near sewage
- not keeping clean.

The Romans did not know why these things caused bad health. But when they built a house or an army camp, they made sure to keep away from bad and dirty places. They also tried to clean up the towns and cities.

Source C

The new Anio aqueduct is taken from the river which is muddy because of the ploughed fields on either side. Because of this water is filtered at the start of the aqueduct.

▲ Julius Frontinus, the Curator of Rome's water supply, writing about AD 100.

Source D

There should be no marshes near buildings. Marshes give off poisonous vapours during the summer. At this time they give birth to animals with mischief-making stings.

▲ Written by Columella, a Roman writer, who lived in the 1st century AD. He was a soldier who became a farmer and writer of books on country life.

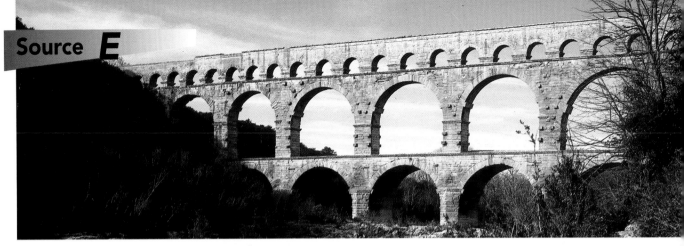

▲ The Pont du Gard aqueduct, which carried water from Uzes to the Roman town at Nîmes in southern France.

Source **F**

We must take care in choosing springs [from which to pipe water].

If a spring runs free and open, look carefully at the people who live nearby before beginning to pipe the water. If they are strong and well then the water is good.

▲ Vitruvius, a Roman writer and architect who lived in the 1st century BC.

Source **G**

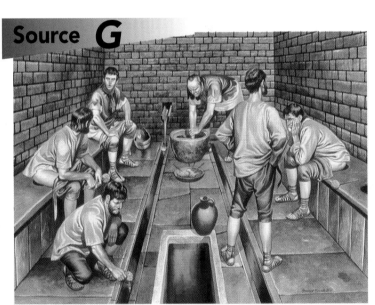

▲ A modern artist's reconstruction of toilets on Hadrian's Wall. Water ran through a channel under the seats to wash away the sewage.

Source **H**

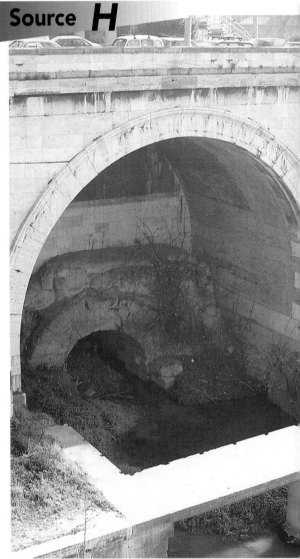

▲ The smaller inner arch is the original outlet of Rome's main sewer into the River Tiber. From the water to the top of the arch is over two metres.

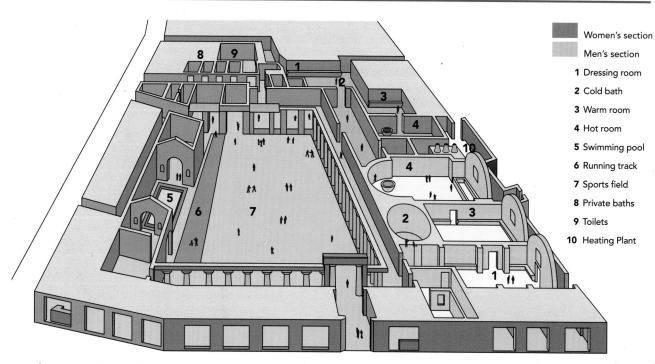

Legend:
- Women's section
- Men's section

1 Dressing room
2 Cold bath
3 Warm room
4 Hot room
5 Swimming pool
6 Running track
7 Sports field
8 Private baths
9 Toilets
10 Heating Plant

▲ **Stabian Baths at Pompeii.**

Aqueducts

The Romans built aqueducts to bring water to towns. There were fourteen aqueducts bringing water to Rome from the hills around the city. There were no pumps so all the aqueducts ran gently down the hill to the city. The water was used for baths, cooking and other things.

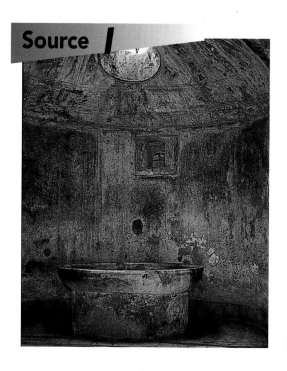

Source 1

◄ **The warm room of the men's section of the Stabian Baths.**

 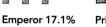 Emperor 17.1%

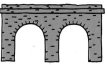 Private houses and industry 38.6%

Military barracks 2.9%

 Official buildings 24.1%

Public buildings, baths and theatres 3.9%

 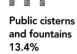 Public cisterns and fountains 13.4%

▲ **The way Rome's water supply was used in AD 100.**

THE FORUM PUBLIC TOILETS, POMPEII

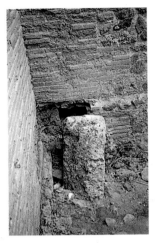

▲ The area marked 'a' on the plan.

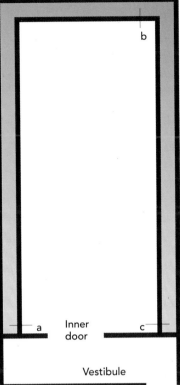

◀ A plan of the Forum public toilet (not to scale).

b

a | Inner door | c

Vestibule

Entrance

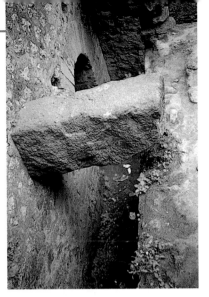

▲ The area marked 'b' on the plan.

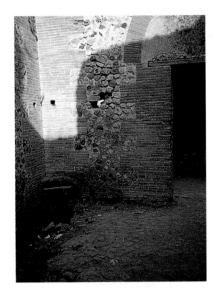

▲ The area marked 'c' on the plan.

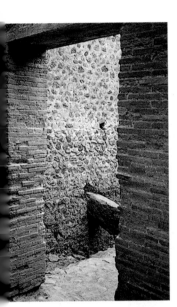

▲ Looking inside from the vestibule.

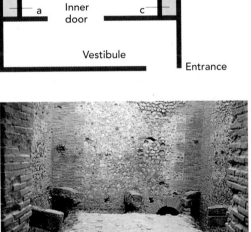

▲ The view from the inner door.

Compare these toilets with the artist's impression of the toilets on Hadrian's Wall (Source G on page 33).

What do a, b and c on this plan show?

How are the two toilets the same?

How are they different?

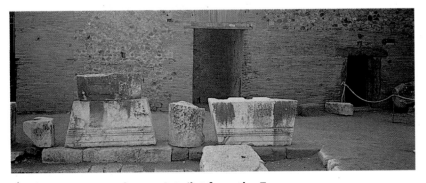

▲ The entrance to the men's toilet from the Forum.

Roman toilets

Roman towns had lots of public toilets. Rome on its own had 150! People did not see going to the toilet as a private thing. There were no separate cubicles. People sat and chatted.

Roman baths

Bathing was even more sociable. A bath house had hot, warm and cold baths. It also had a steam room. Bathers could use the gym or have a massage. Men and women had separate bath houses. If there was only one bath house they used it on different days.

The poor

The poor in the cities were not as lucky as the rich. They did not have running water piped to their homes. They also did not have toilets with pipes which drained into the sewers. They used chamber pots instead, which they sometimes emptied in the street. So not all Roman streets were clean and healthy.

VITRUVIUS

Marcus Vitruvius Pollio lived in the 1st century BC. He was an architect and engineer.

Vitruvius wrote a series of 10 books about architecture, which were called *De architectura*. He wanted to pass on Greek architectural ideas. The books cover:

city planning

building materials

temple building

public buildings (temples and baths)

private buildings

floors and decoration

hydraulics

clocks, measuring and astronomy

civil and military machines.

5.4 The army

It was especially important to keep Roman soldiers healthy. Soldiers with good medical skills looked after other soldiers on the battlefield. There were army hospitals. Army camps were built in healthy places. They were kept clean. Permanent bases, such as forts, often had bath houses, toilets and sewage disposal.

▶ **Vegetius, a Roman writer in the 4th century AD.**

Source J

Soldiers must not remain too long near unhealthy marshes.

A soldier who must face the cold without proper clothing is not in a state to have good health or to march.

He must not drink swamp water.

The generals believe daily exercise is better for soldiers than doctors.

5.5 Galen

Galen's life

AD **129** Born in Pergamum.
Grew up and trained as a doctor at the temple of Asclepios. Went to Alexandria to study.

AD **157** Returned to Pergamum. Became doctor to the gladiators. He was able to see inside the body because of the wounds suffered by the gladiators.

AD **161** Went to Rome and became famous. He told everyone how good he was.

AD **169** Was given the job of doctor to the Emperor's son. From then on he wrote many books.

Galen as a doctor

Galen was a good doctor. Like Hippocrates, Galen said that a doctor must watch his patient carefully (clinical observation). He must write down all the symptoms of an illness.

The four humours and the idea of opposites

Galen used the theory of the four humours and the need to keep the patient in balance. He based a lot of his treatments on opposites. So, if a woman came to him with the symptoms of a cold, he would give a treatment which included pepper or ginger or other warming herbs.

Galen and human anatomy

When Galen was in Alexandria he had studied human skeletons. But he had not been able to dissect human bodies. By his time dissection was forbidden for religious reasons.

Source K

Part of Galen's experiment on a pig to show the importance of the spinal cord.

The animal which you vivisect should not be old – so that it will be easy for you to cut through the vertebrae.

If you cut by the thoracic vertebrae then the first thing that happens is that you see the animal's breathing and voice have been damaged.

If you cut through between the fifth vertebra of the head, then both arms are paralysed.

▲ From *On Anatomical Procedures*, written by Galen in the late 2nd century AD.

However, back in Pergamum and Rome, Galen and other doctors could not even study human skeletons.

How could doctors learn about the human body?

Galen suggested that they should keep a look out for human bones – in cemeteries or after a hanging when a body had been left out to rot.

Galen and animals

Galen learnt as much as he could from dissecting animals. He said barbary apes were most like humans. He also dissected pigs. Using animals gave him problems with things like the brain. He said the brain had a network of blood vessels on the underside. He based a lot of his ideas on this. However, this network is only found in some animals. It is not found in humans.

Why was Galen so important?

Galen was very important for a number of reasons.

1 He wrote over 100 medical books. Most of the books survived. Just having his ideas known about made him important.
2 He developed the ideas of Hippocrates and other great doctors.
3 From these ideas, he developed a complete theory of medicine. He wrote about how the human body works and what happens when it goes wrong. This was very helpful to doctors for hundreds of years.
4 He lived at a time when the Romans still believed in many gods. But he often wrote about 'the creator' or the great designer of the human body. This meant that Christians and Muslims, who only believed in one god, accepted his ideas. In fact, Galen's ideas dominated medicine in Europe for the next 1,300 years.

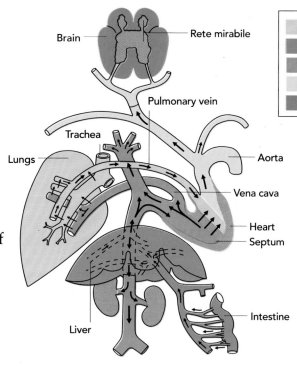

▲ **Galen's physiological system.**

Pneuma (life-giving spirit) breathed in. Went from the lungs to the heart to mix with the blood.

Chyle (the goodness from food) went from the intestines to the liver. Made into blood with Natural Spirit.

Blood with Natural Spirit went throughout the body nourishing and enabling growth. From the heart some went to the lungs, and some passed through the septum to mix with the pneuma to form blood with Vital Spirit.

Blood with Vital Spirit went into the arteries giving power to the body. It was changed into blood with Animal Spirit at the brain.

Blood with Animal Spirit went through the nerves (which Galen believed were hollow) to give the body sensation and motion.

Diagram labels: Brain, Rete mirabile, Pulmonary vein, Trachea, Lungs, Aorta, Vena cava, Heart, Septum, Intestine, Liver

Legend: pneuma / chyle / blood with natural spirit / blood with vital spirit / blood with animal spirit

COMMODUS

Commodus was emperor of Rome from AD 177 to AD 192. Galen was his personal doctor from AD 169 onwards.

Commodus ruled jointly with his father for the first three years of his reign. When his father died he soon became hated because he was both cruel and unfair. He also pulled out of the war with the German tribes. The tribes, left to flourish, eventually destroyed the Empire.

Commodus seems to have eventually gone mad. He believed that he was the god Hercules come back to life. He was so convinced of this that he fought lions and gladiators to prove it.

Commodus was assassinated. His madness became so bad that even his friends could take no more of his behaviour. Three of his most trusted supporters, including his mistress, paid for him to be killed.

The Romans didn't just provide clean water, toilets, sewage systems and baths for the rich. They were available for all town dwellers. Not all bath houses were huge complexes like the Stabian Baths shown on page 34. Small communities, or military posts, had small bath houses.

A small provincial city in England, *Durovernum* [Canterbury], had a large public bath and at least one small private one. Destruction of part of the medieval city centre by bombing during the Second World War enabled archaeologists to excavate the small bath house shown here. It is about 16m x 12m, as opposed to the Stabian Baths (66m x 96m).

Source 1

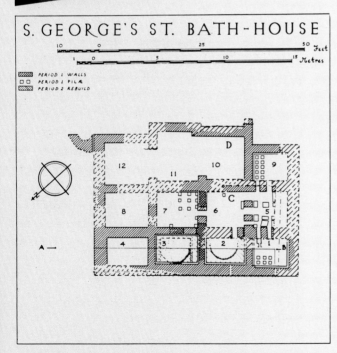

▲ The St George's St. bath house, Canterbury, as it would have been in AD 220–30.

St George's St. bath house
The baths were built in about AD 220–30. They were altered in about AD 360.

AD 220–30
At this time Room 12 was a changing room.
Room 8 was a cold room, with a cold bath off it in Room 4.
Rooms 7 and 6 were warm rooms.
Rooms 2 and 3 had warm basins.
Room 5 was a hot room.
Rooms 1 and 9 had hot baths.

CHAPTER 6

THE FALL OF THE ROMAN EMPIRE IN THE WEST

The Roman Empire – East and West

By the 4th century AD the Roman Empire was weak. It split into two. The Eastern Empire was ruled from Byzantium. The Western Empire was ruled from Rome. But soon Rome was invaded by tribes from other parts of Europe, such as the Huns, Goths and Vandals. Britain was invaded by the Anglo-Saxons.

What the fall of the Roman Empire meant

The Romans left Britain in about AD 410. All over the Roman Empire government had been strong. There had been good roads, big towns, clean water systems, sewage systems and strong laws so people felt safe. When the Romans became weak all this broke down. No one mended the roads or the water pipes. The towns fell down. The laws broke down. People did not feel safe. Local kings tried to keep some sort of law and order but there was a lot of fighting. People went back to living in mud huts and growing their own food.

The loss of learning

Within a hundred years no one was left who knew how to build stone roads, aqueducts, bridges or public baths. Libraries fell down. Books were lost. People could not learn about medicine, mathematics or anything else. Historians often called this period of time in Western Europe, the **Dark Ages**.

Source A

Snapped rooftrees, towers fallen, the work of Giants, the stonesmiths, mouldereth.

And the wielders and wrights [workmen]? Earthgrip holds them – gone, long gone, fast in gravesgrasp.

▲ Part of an Anglo-Saxon poem, *The Ruin*. It describes a ruined Roman city.

Source B

When you see a dung beetle digging, catch it and some earth. Wave it about and say:

Remedium facio ad ventris dolorum [help stomach ache].

Then throw the beetle away, over your back, without looking.

When someone comes to you with stomach ache, hold the stomach between your hands. They will be well. This will work for a year after catching the beetle.

▲ A Saxon cure for stomach ache, around the 6th century AD.

Catch a frog when neither moon or sun is shining. Cut off the hind legs. Wrap them in deerskin. Put the frog's left leg to the patient's gouty left foot and he will certainly be cured.

▲ **A cure used by 'Gilbert', a doctor working in the early 11th century.**

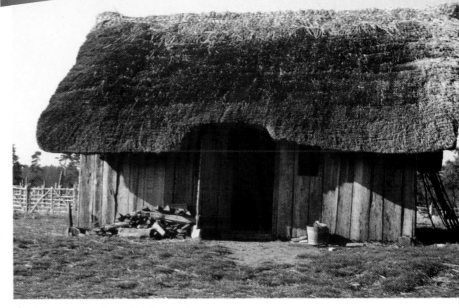

▼ **The Dark Ages timeline.**

▲ **A reconstruction of a Saxon home.**

AD 350   AD 400   AD 500   AD 600   AD 700   AD 800   AD 900   AD 1000   AD 1050

Last Western Roman Emperor overthrown

The Ruin written

'Gilbert' working as a doctor

Fall of Rome to the Goths

Last Roman troops leave Britain

Roman Empire spilt into two

GILDAS

Gildas 'the Wise' (c AD 500 – c AD 572) was a monk who lived in Britain and Brittany (France) during the Dark Ages. He believed that the Saxon invasions were a punishment from God for the sins of the wicked Britons.

Gildas wrote one of the few books to survive from this time. It was called *On the Ruin of Britain*. He spends most of the book telling the British that their sins have caused all their troubles.

Gildas also tells the story of a British leader (Ambrosius) who beat the Saxons at the battle of Badon Hill. Some people think that Ambrosius is the person that the stories about King Arthur have been based on.

PROGRESS AND REGRESS

In this book we are looking at one aspect of human society, medicine, through time. We need to be careful how we use the technical words which describe the story. **Progress** means something moving forward. In our context this means getting better, improving. **Regress** means something moving backwards, in our case, getting worse.

CHAPTER 7

ORIENTAL MEDICINE — ISLAM AND CHINA

7.1 Islamic civilization

The Roman Empire in the West had collapsed by about AD 500. Soon a new empire grew up. It was based on the teachings of Muhammad who was born in Arabia in AD 570. By AD 1000 all the area shown on the map below was united by Muhammad's religion (**Islam**) and by speaking Arabic.

The religion of Islam

The Holy Book of Islam is the *Qur'an*. It is all the teachings of Muhammad written down. The *Qur'an* says how a follower of Muhammad should live. A follower of Muhammad is called a Muslim. The *Qur'an* tells people what to do and eat on special days. It tells everyone how to behave. This includes how parents should treat their children and how the rich should treat the poor.

The rule of the Abbasids

The **Abbasids** ruled the Arabic Empire from the city of Baghdad. They were descended from Muhammad's uncle. They ruled for about 500 years.

The city of Baghdad

The Abbasids built the city of Baghdad. It had lots of fine buildings and public baths. The city was the centre of a huge empire. It was wealthy because it traded with many countries, such as China, India, Russia and Africa.

Muslims settle in new lands

Muslims settled in new countries shown on the map. Wherever they went they built schools and **mosques**. Later they built universities.

MUHAMMAD

Muhammad (AD 570–632) was born in Mecca, in modern Saudi Arabia.

Muhammad started a new religion, Islam. This spread rapidly over the Middle East and beyond. The Islamic religion had rules that affected all parts of people's lives, including their medical practices.

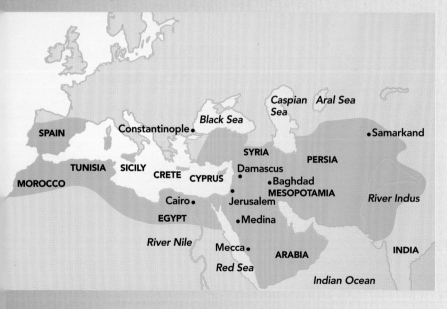

▲ Countries which were part of the Arabic Empire in about AD 1000.

Greek and Roman learning lived on

The Roman Empire in the West collapsed. But Greek and Roman learning lived on in the East.

Who lived in the Arabic Empire?

The Arabic Empire had many different people living in it. They did not all share the same religion. Some were followers of Islam. Some were Jews. Others were Christians, like Nestorius. The two things that united them were using the Arab language and living in the Arabic Empire.

Nestorius in the 5th century AD

Nestorius was a Christian who lived in Persia. He and his followers translated some of the Greek and Roman medical books into Arabic.

Hunain ibn Ishaq

Hunain ibn Ishaq (known as Johannitius) brought Greek and Roman medical books to Baghdad. Some of these books were by Hippocrates. Others were by Galen. He translated them into Arabic. About 300 years later these books reached Europe and were translated from Arabic into Latin. This was how European doctors in the Middle Ages learnt about Greek medicine.

Source B

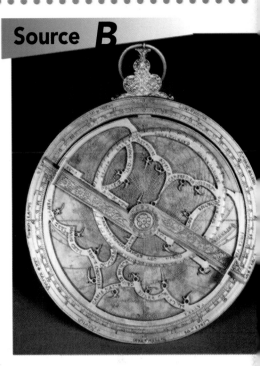

▶ The astrolabe. It was probably invented by a Greek in about 150 BC. It was used to navigate at sea. This one dates from the 16th century AD.

How Greek and Roman ideas survived
Learning continued in the East. ↓ Greek medical books translated into Arabic. ↓ Medical books later taken to Western Europe and translated into Latin.

Source A

In the 9th and 10th centuries, Cordoba was a city of 200,000 houses, 600 mosques and 900 public baths. Its library had 600,000 books.

▲ Hugh Thomas, *Spain*, 1964.

DISCORIDES

Discorides (c AD 40–90) was a surgeon in the Roman army. He also wrote a book about herbal cures, *De Materia Medica*. Doctors used his book for over 1,000 years.

Causes of disease

In Muhammad's time many Arab doctors said that evil spirits made people ill. Some Arab doctors, who read the Greek and Roman medical books, decided to try some of these ideas. They used the ideas they thought worked, such as the idea of the four humours.

Rhazes (about AD 900)

Rhazes was a Persian. He was an important doctor in Baghdad in about AD 900. He used the idea of the humours. He also used the idea of observation or watching closely. He was the first doctor to write about the difference between measles and **smallpox**.

Avicenna (AD 980–1037)

Avicenna was a very important doctor. He wrote a book about medicine. It was called the *Canon of Medicine*. Avicenna used the ideas of Galen. He also added some of his own.

Why was Avicenna's book so important?

Avicenna's book was very important. First, it is a very good book about disease and medicine. Second, the book was translated into Latin. This meant that doctors in Europe could read it. So they learnt about the ideas of Galen which had been forgotten in Europe. *The Canon of Medicine* was the main book for training doctors until about 1700.

Source C

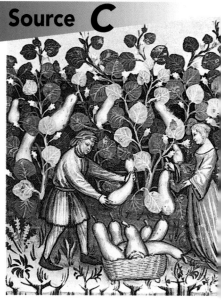

▲ A medieval European picture showing people harvesting marrows which were used to cleanse the bowels and quench thirst. This was a good example of how Arabic manuscripts were used in the West.

AVICENNA

Avicenna (AD 980–1037), whose Arabic name was Ibn Fina, studied law as well as medicine. He became famous as a surgeon. He travelled with the Persian army when it went to war. Avicenna gave lessons in surgery and also wrote books, even while he was travelling with the army. He even wrote books when he was put in prison by the enemies of Persia! His books influenced western doctors for centuries.

Source D

Smallpox brings backache, fever, stinging pains, red cheeks and eyes and difficulty with breathing.

There is more excitement, sickness and unrest in measles than in smallpox. Aching in the back is less.

▲ From *On Smallpox and Measles*, written by Rhazes, a Persian doctor, in about AD 900.

Hospitals

By AD 850 Baghdad had its first hospital and by AD 931, doctors had to pass examinations. Other hospitals were set up all over the Arabic Empire. The most famous hospitals were at Damascus and Cairo.

Surgery

The greatest surgeon was Albucasis who was born in Spain in about AD 936. He was a careful man. He told surgeons to work out what they were going to do before they cut into someone. He wrote about amputations, taking stones out of the bladder, setting broken bones and many other operations. He also wrote about sewing wounds up.

Following what Galen said

Islamic law said that Arab doctors must not dissect human bodies. This meant that the Arab doctors could not check up on what Galen had said. One doctor who disagreed with Galen was Ibn an-Nafis. In 1242 he said that blood did not pass through the septum (see page 38). He was right and Galen was wrong. The ideas of Ibn an-Nafis did not spread to Europe and people continued to believe in Galen.

Chemistry

The Arabs invented new ways of making medicines. This also helped some drugs to be more widely used. These included senna, musk and camphor.

Source E

In the Cairo hospital there were special places for the wounded, for eye patients and for those with fever. There were fountains in their rooms to keep them cool. When the patient left the hospital, he was given five pieces of gold, so that he did not have to go back to work at once.

▲ W. J. Bishop, *The Early History of Surgery*, 1960.

Source F

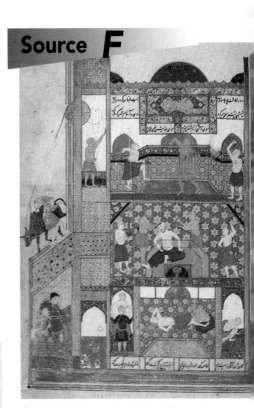

▲ Caliph Manum having a shower, haircut and massage in the bath-house of his palace in Baghdad.

ALBUCASIS

Abul Kasim, known as Albucasis (c AD 936–1013), was born in Spain. He was the Spanish caliph's doctor.

Albucasis wrote a book called *On Surgery*. It was based on the work of earlier doctors and his own observation.

China was a long way from India, the Islamic Empire and Europe. China developed its own civilization and type of medicine.

The history of China

From early in China's history there were some very strong emperors. There were also times when there was civil war and China broke up into separate parts.

Strong government

However, over hundreds of years the emperors set up a very strong government. There were thousands of civil servants in the main cities and all over China. They collected taxes, ran the law courts, ran the army, ran the flood and irrigation works (that controlled the rivers) and ran many of the industries.

The Silk Road

The Silk Road was the route to India and the Arabic Empire. It went through deserts and over mountains for hundreds of miles. Goods such as silk and paper came from China to India and the West. Ideas also spread this way. Chinese inventions including windmills, gunpowder and wheelbarrows came to the West. In return China got ideas such as **Buddhism** from India. It also obtained some ideas on medicine from India. (India had its own very old tradition of medicine called **Ayurvedic** medicine.)

Source G

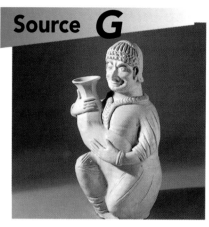

▲ A pottery figure of a foreign merchant. The Chinese found the round eyes, big noses and light hair of people from the West both ugly and fascinating. They looked down on anyone from outside China.

FIRST EMPEROR

The First Emperor united China. He had the Great Wall of China built. He took all kinds of drugs and medicines, hoping they would help him live forever. They probably killed him in the end.

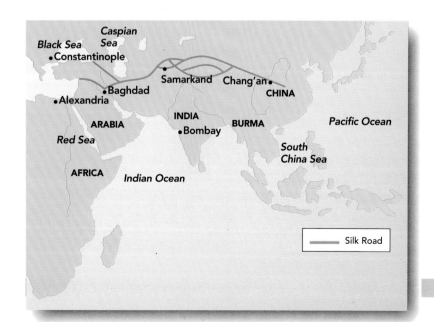

◄ The Silk Road. All the goods carried along the Silk Road were carried by camels, through deserts and over mountains.

Keeping well is keeping in balance

Greek medicine looked at the balance of the humours in the body. Arabic medicine used the same ideas. They took these ideas to India, where the Indians already had a system of medicine that said a person was well if everything was in balance. The Chinese had similar ideas about balance. They talked about Yin and Yang.

Yin and Yang

In Chinese medicine, ourselves and everything around us are a balance of Yin and Yang. Below is a diagram to give you an idea of what Yin and Yang mean.

	Yang
Yang = hot, day, sunshine, busy. Yin = cool, night, shade, rest.	
	Yin

Chinese doctors said that everyone must live in balance. In the day we are busy. In the night we rest. If a person is busy all the time, he or she will become ill.

The aim of Chinese medicine

The aim of Chinese medicine is to keep a balance between Yin and Yang in the body. To do this doctors advise about food and exercise. They use herbs and **acupuncture** to bring a sick person back into balance. (Not too hot. Not too cold. Not too busy. Not too tired).

Acupuncture and moxibustion

Acupuncture is putting fine needles into points on the body to balance the energy or *qi* (pronounced 'chi' in Chinese).

Source H

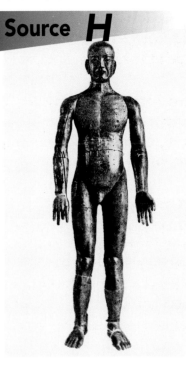

▶ This bronze man shows all the common acupuncture points. They are pinholes. For examinations the figure was covered with wax and filled with water. Students had to know where the points were. They put needles through the wax. If they were in the right place they pierced the wax and water spurted out of the holes.

This *qi* flows round the body. It can become blocked in some way. The needles make the qi flow well. This brings Yin and Yang back into balance.

Thousands of books have been written about Chinese medicine. Most Chinese doctors use a mixture of herbal cures and acupuncture.

HUA TO

Hua To (AD 115–205) was a famous surgeon. He is said to have been one of the first surgeons to use anaesthetics. He gave his patients a secret powder mixed with wine. This made them sleepy and also made them numb so they felt less pain.

CHAPTER 8

MEDICINE IN THE MIDDLE AGES

8.1 Western Europe in the Middle Ages

When the Roman Empire broke up Europe became divided into many small countries. The Christian religion was the only thing these countries had in common. They all looked up to the Pope as head of the Christian Church. All the church services were in Latin – the language the Romans had used.

For 400 years Europe muddled along. Then some countries, such as England, became more united and stronger. Islamic countries in the Middle East also became stronger. The Christians were afraid of the power of Islam. This led to wars (known as the **Crusades**) between Christians and Islam.

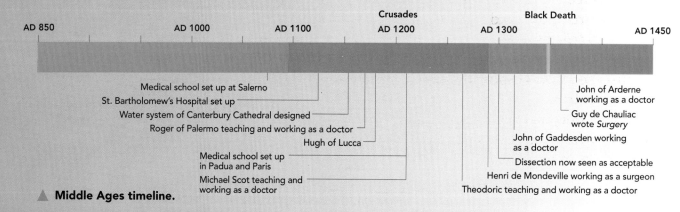

| AD 850 | AD 1000 | AD 1100 | Crusades AD 1200 | AD 1300 | Black Death | AD 1450 |

Medical school set up at Salerno
St. Bartholomew's Hospital set up
Water system of Canterbury Cathedral designed
Roger of Palermo teaching and working as a doctor
Hugh of Lucca
Medical school set up in Padua and Paris
Michael Scot teaching and working as a doctor

John of Arderne working as a doctor
Guy de Chauliac wrote *Surgery*
John of Gaddesden working as a doctor
Dissection now seen as acceptable
Henri de Mondeville working as a surgeon
Theodoric teaching and working as a doctor

▲ **Middle Ages timeline.**

8.2 Beliefs about the causes of disease

Beliefs about the causes of disease in the Middle Ages

1 Some people believed that magic and evil spirits caused disease.

2 Some people believed that the planets caused disease.

3 Some people, like monks, used the theory of the four humours to look for the cause of disease.

4 The Church said that God sometimes sent disease to punish a person.

Source A

I allowed only red things to be about his bed, by which I cured him, without leaving a trace of the smallpox pustules on him.

▲ **Written by John of Gaddesden, Edward II's doctor, in 1314. He is describing how he had cured Edward's son of smallpox.**

Source B

For scrofula tumours and boils, use the herb scelerat softened and mixed with pig dung.

◀ From a 13th century medical book. Scrofula was a form of tuberculosis.

Treatments

1 Sometimes magical cures were used. For instance, a herbal drink with a bitter taste might drive out an evil spirit.
2 Some doctors carried a book about the planets around with them, to help them discover what was wrong with their patients. This book was called a *Vademecum*. It had charts to show how to tell what was wrong by looking at the sick person's urine. It also told how and when to bleed a patient.
3 Some monks and some doctors used herbs to treat disease. They worked to get the sick person's body back into balance again.
4 Many people prayed to God for help. Some went on **pilgrimages** to places like Canterbury to ask the saints to help them get well.

Source C

When scrofula comes to a head cut so that the pus comes out. If they harden for a month or more, or if the patient is a boy use this oil.

At the declining of the moon make eleven poultices of iris and soft radish, use one a day. Bleed the patient at least once.

If all this is not sufficient, surgery must be used. Hold the patient's throat, cut the skin and pull the scrofula out with a hook.

▲ From a 14th century book by the doctor, Roger of Salerno.

JOHN OF GADDESDEN

John of Gaddesden (1280–1361) studied medicine at Montpellier, France.

He was the best known doctor in England. He was probably the person that the doctor in Chaucer's *Canterbury Tales* was based on.

John was the royal doctor. He also wrote a medical book, *Rosa Anglica*. It had no new ideas in it, but it summed up old ones.

Source D

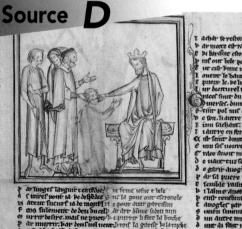

◀ **Edward the Confessor touches a man to cure him from scrofula. Many kings and queens of England were believed to be able to cure scrofula.**

The Romans left Britain in the 5th century. For the next few hundred years Europe muddled along. By about AD 1000 things began to change.

Teaching doctors

The first medical school was at **Salerno** in Italy. The teachers used the books of Hippocrates and Galen. (Many of these books had been saved by the Arab doctors. Now they were translated back into Latin). The use of these books led to three things.

- Teachers began to teach clinical observation again.
- Teachers began to teach more about keeping clean again.
- Teachers began to teach the theory of the four humours again.

However, the books of Hippocrates and Galen were the only books used. Young doctors were taught that everything in them was true.

Higher standards

The Holy Roman Emperor was very impressed by the teaching at Salerno. So, in 1221 he passed a law saying that only doctors trained there could treat patients. This only applied to rich people who were sick! However, it was the first time that some standard was fixed for training doctors.

Other medical schools

Other medical schools started, such as Bologna and Paris. By the l4th century there were many places in Europe where doctors could train. More and more doctors were trained. Some began to question the ideas of Hippocrates and Galen. New ideas were put forward. One of these was using the colour of urine to help to diagnose what was happening to a sick person. Even the Christian Church moved with the times. Doctors were allowed to see dissection done so that they could learn more about the human body.

Source E

When you are asked if a sick person will get better or die, look at his star sign.

Also examine the moon for the sick person because it can tell us something too.

Then check the tenth house and its ruling sign, since they signify health and medicine.

Do the same for the sixth house, since they signify illness. Then the eighth house, since they signify death for the sick. Then see the fourth house and its lord, since this signifies the end of all the others.

▲ From a book by Michael Scot, a teacher at the medical school in Salerno.

Urine and health

One of the most widely accepted of the new ideas was that the colour and smell of urine could help diagnose sickness. Urine should be clear, pale yellow and not smelly. Strong sweet smells or ammonia smells were a bad sign. So was a dark or cloudy colour.

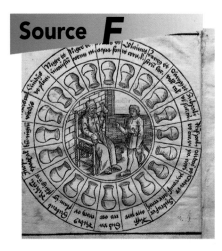

Source **F**

▲ A urine chart from 1506. They were in use much earlier. The use of the colour of urine to diagnose disease was a new idea that became widely accepted.

8.4 Ordinary people

Rich people

The books of Hippocrates and Galen were still the main books that teachers used in the medical schools. The doctors who trained at the medical schools treated rich people. So only the rich came into contact with the ideas of Hippocrates and Galen, or any of the new ideas.

Ordinary people in the country

Most people lived in the country. They were not rich. If they were ill they went on treating themselves and their families as they had done for hundreds of years. They used herbs or magical cures. Sometimes there were women and men in the village who had learnt about herbs and healing. Often sick people turned to them for help. These people did not write anything down so we do not know much about them.

Women

There is some evidence that the medical school at Salerno trained women as well as men. However, more and more women were being pushed out of medicine. They were only really accepted as **midwives** and healers.

Source **G**

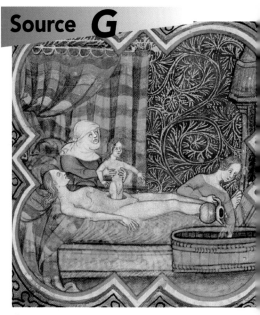

▲ A woman delivering a baby by Caesarean section.

Barber-surgeons and surgeons

Barber-surgeons cut people's hair. They also did some surgery. They often learnt from their fathers and were the only sort of surgeons that poor people could afford.

Surgeons had medical training. But the job of a surgeon was hard work and very messy. Most doctors did not want to be surgeons. So there were few well trained surgeons in the Middle Ages.

Learning surgery

Look at Source I. By about 1300 dissection was allowed in medical schools. In this picture the teacher is reading from a book on the human body by Galen. His assistant is cutting up the body. The assistant's job was to find the things that were in Galen's book.

If he did not find the things Galen wrote about then the teacher said he had messed up the dissection. Galen could not be wrong.

Source I

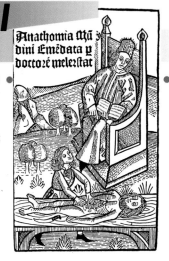

A lecturer reads from a book while his assistant dissects a body.

Pain and infection

Pain and infection were the main problems of surgery. One or two surgeons tried to dull the pain with drugs. (see Source K). Others tried to deal with infection by washing wounds in wine. (We now know this is an antiseptic). Nothing seems to have worked well enough for all surgeons to use it.

Successful operations

Like the Egyptians, Greeks, Romans and Arabs, the surgeons of the Middle Ages found that the only successful operations were minor ones on the outside of the body. So mending broken bones and setting dislocations, removing cataracts and small cysts were successful. Digging deep into the body usually meant death.

Source H

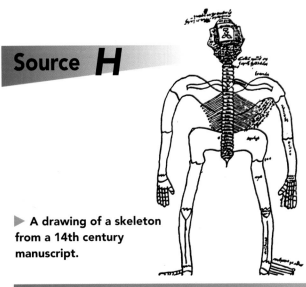

▶ A drawing of a skeleton from a 14th century manuscript.

Source J

It is dangerous for a surgeon who is not famous to operate in any new way.

▲ Written by Henri de Mondeville (1260–1320), a master surgeon at the University of Bologna.

Take the gall of a boar, and three spoonfuls each of juice of hemlock, wild briony, lettuce, opium poppy, henbane and vinegar.

Mix together and add three spoonfuls of the mixture to a bottle of wine or ale.

The man to be operated on should drink the whole bottle by a warm fire. He will fall asleep and then can be operated on.

▲ A recipe for an anaesthetic from John of Arderne, a well-known English surgeon in 1376.

MONDINO DE LUZZI

Mondino de Luzzi (c 1270–1326) was the most important anatomist of the Middle Ages. He worked at the University of Bologna. By the end of the 14th century this was seen as the leading medical school in Europe.

Mondino had read the work of Arab anatomists, so he knew about their discoveries. They also told him about the work of Galen. Mondino's book *Anatomy* was written in 1316. It dominated the teaching of anatomy in Europe for the next 200 years.

Mondino did his own dissections as part of his lectures on anatomy at the university. He stressed the importance of dissecting humans, not animals, when studying human anatomy.

8.6 Public health

The Romans had been very well organized. They had piped clean water to the towns. This had made it easy for people to keep clean.

But in the Middle Ages governments were not as well organized as the Romans. So there was not much clean water in towns.

Towns

In the Middle Ages towns were run by groups of men who formed a local council. They raised money to run the town.

Usually there was not enough money to pipe water to everyone, or to make drains to take the dirty water away.

The lane called Ebbegate used to be a right of way until it was closed up by Thomas at Wytte and William de Hockele who built latrines which stuck out from the walls of the houses. From these latrines human filth falls out onto the heads of passers-by.

▲ Evidence given in a court case heard in London, in 1321.

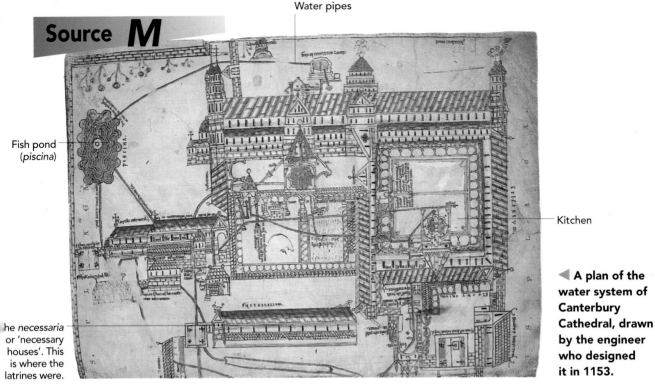

Water pipes

Fish pond
(*piscina*)

Kitchen

he *necessaria* or 'necessary houses'. This is where the latrines were.

◀ **A plan of the water system of Canterbury Cathedral, drawn by the engineer who designed it in 1153.**

What happened to the rubbish and sewage?

Sometimes people built toilets over a stream or even had a cesspit under the house. Streams clogged up with sewage and stank. **Cesspits** overflowed. Some people put their rubbish and sewage in the street. Councils sometimes passed laws against this but no one took much notice. The only time that people cleaned up was when serious disease broke out.

Monasteries

Monasteries were often rich and well organized. They often piped clean water from a river and built drains to take the sewage far from the monastery. Canterbury Cathedral (also a monastery) had a complicated water system.

The water from the river was piped through five tanks to make sure it was clean. Water from washing was used to flush the toilets which were built away from the main buildings. Monks washed their hands and faces before meals and at other times.

All the streets are so badly paved that they get wet easily. This happens a lot because of the cattle carrying water, and the rain. Evil smelling mud is formed which seems to last all year round.

▲ **Written by a visitor to Winchester in 1286.**

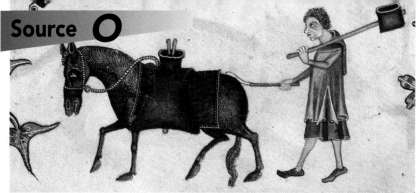

Source O

▲ An illustration of a water seller, from the 14th century *Lutterell Psalter*.

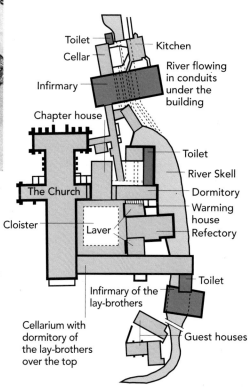

▲ Fountains Abbey, a monastery in Yorkshire, showing the water supply and drainage.

Hospitals

By about 1200 there were a few hospitals in Europe. Most were set up by monks. Not all of them had doctors or surgeons. They did not treat sickness. They just made the patients as comfortable as they could. Apart from this there were a few hospitals for **lepers** (people suffering from leprosy), and other hospitals for women having babies.

8.7 The Black Death

The Black Death: 1347–49

The Black Death was also called the **plague**. It came to Europe in 1347. Within a year it had reached Britain. People fell ill with a temperature and soon lumps (buboes) appeared in the armpit or groin. The buboes went black. After a few days the person either died or began to get better.

What caused the Black Death?

We now know there were two main sorts of plague. Pneumonic plague was spread by coughs and sneezing. Bubonic plague was caused by flea bites. The fleas lived on black rats. Rats were common in the dirty towns and on the ships of that time. The fleas spread quickly from the rats to other animals and then to people.

BRADWARDINE

Thomas Bradwardine (c 1290–1349) studied at Oxford University. He was a very good mathematician and astronomer.

Bradwardine was chosen to become Archbishop of Canterbury while he was away in Europe. As soon as he heard the news he hurried back to England.

Bradwardine landed on 19 August 1349 and headed for London. He caught the plague as soon as he arrived in London. He died on 26 August.

What did people at the time think?

No one at the time knew what caused the plague. The sources below show some of the things people thought caused it.

None of the reasons given, however, fully explained how the plague was spread.

How many people died?

No one knew how to stop the plague. In 1348 and 1349, between one third and one half of the population of Britain died. As many as 2.5 million people might have died from the disease. Sometimes whole villages were wiped out.

Source P

Some people believed the cause of the Black Death was poison. It was either the Jews, or cripples or nobles poisoning people. If someone was carrying a powder or ointment people made him swallow it for fear it might be poisonous.

But the truth is that there were two causes. The general cause was the close position of the three great planets, Saturn, Jupiter and Mars on 24th March 1345, in the 14th degree of Aquarius. The particular cause in each person was the state of the body – bad digestion, weakness or blockage.

▲ From *On Surgery*, written in 1363, by Guy de Chauliac a French doctor.

Source R

Whoever touched the sick or dead was infected and died. I, waiting for death 'till it come, have put these things in writing.

▲ An Irish friar who died from the Black Death in 1349.

Source S

The plague comes from the ground or the air or both together.

As we see a privy [toilet] which makes the air dirty next to a chamber.

Sometimes it comes from dead bodies or stagnant water.

▲ Written in 1485 by the Bishop of Aarhus in Denmark.

Source Q

Many people think that the Jews did not poison the water. They only confessed because they were tortured.

Wise people think the plague was caused by an earthquake which let out bad vapours into the springs and wells. Many Jews are doctors and know how to avoid the plague.

▲ From a book about the history of Switzerland by Glig Tshudi, written in about 1560. He used many reports from 1349.

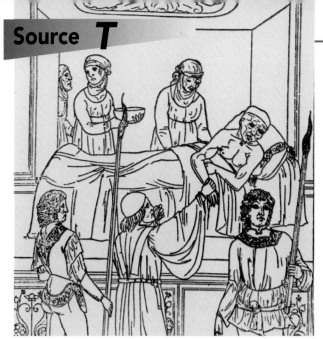

A doctor with a plague victim. He is carrying a pomander to keep off bad smells. His assistants carry tapers to clear bad air.

GUY DE CHAULIAC

Guy de Chauliac (c 1300–68) was a French doctor and surgeon. He was the Pope's personal doctor for a while. He caught the plague during the 1348 outbreak, but lived.

Chauliac wrote a book on surgery called *Chirurgia Magna*. It was published in 1363 and became one of the most important books on surgery to be written at the time.

Chauliac wrote about things other than surgery. He talked about caring for teeth and replacing missing teeth with pieces of bone. He was one of the first doctors to use weights to extend broken legs.

Cures

People in the Middle Ages could not stop the plague from spreading. They could not treat it. However, they tried both spiritual and physical cures.

Source **U**

The filth lying in the streets of the city and its suburbs must be removed with all speed to places far distant.

The city and suburbs are to be kept clean so that no further deaths may arise from such smells.

An order sent by King Edward III to the Lord Mayor of London, in 1349.

Source **V**

The swellings should be softened with figs and cooked onions mixed with yeast and butter, then opened and treated like ulcers.

From *On Surgery* by Guy de Chauliac.

Source **W**

The reek of plague sores poisons the air because the humours of the body are infected. In times of plague people should not crowd together, because someone may be infected.

Avoid all four stinks – the stable, stinking fields or streets, dead bodies and stinking water. Clean your house. Make a fire. Burn herbs, such as bay and juniper, to clear the air.

Written in 1485 by the Bishop of Aarhus in Denmark.

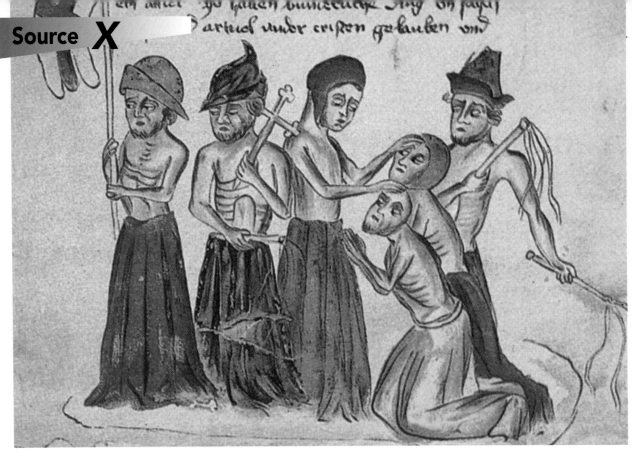

▲ Flagellants whipping themselves. These people thought the Black Death was sent by God because people were sinful.

Source Y

About Michaelmas 1349, over six hundred men came to London from Flanders. They wore clothes from the waist down, but otherwise were bare. They wore a cap with a red cross.

Each had a whip with three tails with nails in them. They marched one behind the other and whipped themselves till they bled.

They were singing and chanting as they went.

They would throw themselves on the ground three times in turn, stretching their arms out like they were on the cross. Then they would take turns whipping the one lying on the ground.

▲ A description of the flagellants in London by a witness.

HOW MANY DIED?

It is very hard to say how many people died during the plague. The careful records of births and deaths that we keep today did not exist at the time. We are not even sure how many people there were in any major European country at the time. People at the time did not know, either. People guessed population numbers. We have no way of knowing how accurate they were.

Guesses from the time about deaths from the plague, combined with as much modern research as possible, suggest that about a third of the population of Europe died between 1347 and 1351.

Medieval Christians believed that saints could intercede with God on their behalf. They also believed that honouring a saint by making an offering to them, or making a pilgrimage to the shrine where the saint was buried (or both), would make prayers more likely to succeed. Pilgrimage became one of the range of possibilities for people who were ill and looking for a cure.

The Church was very careful to be sure that the person chosen to be a saint really deserved it. Any evidence that prayers to a possible saint had produced miraculous cures was carefully investigated. In 1307, Church commissioners went to investigate the shrine of Thomas Cantilupe. Cantilupe (once bishop of Hereford) had died 25 years before. People talked of miracle cures at his shrine. When the commissioners arrived they found people were already making offerings at the shrine, even though Cantilupe was not yet a saint. They found the offerings listed in Source 1.

Two and a half months later, when the commissioners had finished their investigations, they found the offerings had increased by:

3 ships (2 silver and 1 wax)
a silver image of a man
85 wax images of people or limbs
2 children's shifts.

The commissioners did not count coins either time, although they noted that coins were by far the most common offering.

Cantilupe was made a saint in 1320. The range of offerings at famous shrines, like Becket's in Canterbury, would have been a great deal more.

Source 1

170 silver ships

41 wax ships

129 silver images, either of whole bodies or different limbs

436 whole images of men, wax

1,200 wax images of parts of the body and limbs

77 figures of horses, animals and birds

an uncountable quanity of [wax] eyes, breasts, teeth, ears

95 silk and linen children's shifts

108 walking sticks for cripples

3 carts

1 wax cart

10 large square candles

38 clothes of silk and gold

many belts

many ladies' jewels including:

450 gold rings

70 silver rings

65 gold brooches and pins

many precious stones

iron chains offered by prisoners

anchors of ships

lances, spears, swords, knives

CHAPTER 9

MEDICINE IN EARLY MODERN EUROPE

9.1 Renaissance and Reformation

The Middle Ages had been a time of slow change. Between 1430 and 1700 (usually called the **Early Modern** period) things changed more quickly.

Renaissance – from 1430

Renaissance means rebirth. From about 1430 there was a rebirth of old ideas. People looked back to the ideas of the Greeks and Romans. They read Greek and Roman books. They wanted to learn everything the Greeks and Romans had learned. This was the rebirth of interest and learning. They had new ideas, too, about how the world worked. Most of these ideas were based on careful observation.

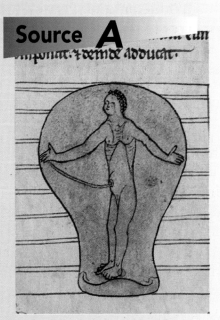

Source A

◀ **A drawing of a foetus from a medieval book for midwives.**

Source B

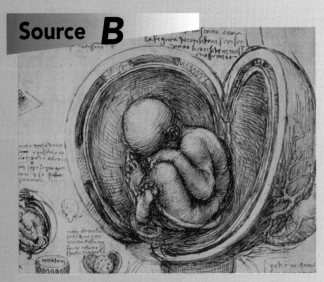

▲ A drawing of a foetus by Leonardo da Vinci. He dissected the body of a woman who died in pregnancy.

Art in the Renaissance

Artists said that pictures had to look real. Artists went to see human bodies dissected so that they knew exactly what a body was like. Some artists drew so well their pictures helped doctors to understand the way bodies were put together.

The Reformation

The **Reformation** went hand in hand with the Renaissance. People read and thought more. They wanted more change. Many people said that the Church was too powerful. They wanted to change the Church.

Printing

In the Middle Ages books were written by hand. They took months or years to make. They were so expensive they were kept chained up in libraries. But **Johannes Gutenberg** changed this. He printed the first books in Europe in 1454. Soon printed books were rolling off the printing presses. Many more people could now read about the ideas of the Greeks and Romans, or the new ideas on medicine and religion.

Medicine

The new printed books, with their clear pictures by famous artists, made a huge difference to medicine. Soon doctors were questioning the old ideas about the human body.

Paracelsus

Paracelsus was typical of the new questioning. He was the town doctor and lecturer at Basel University. In 1527 he invited students, barber-surgeons and anyone who was interested to come and listen to him. He started his first lecture by burning a pile of books. These were books by Galen and Avicenna. Paracelsus said: *'Galen is a liar and a fake. Avicenna (a famous Arab doctor) is a kitchen master. They are good for nothing. You will not need them. Reading never made a doctor. Patients are the only books.'*

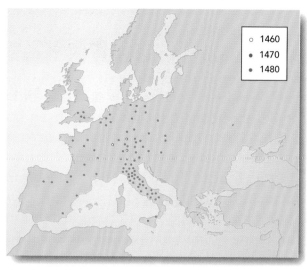

○	1460
●	1470
●	1480

▲ **The spread of printers' workshops, 1460–80.**

LEONARDO DA VINCI

Leonardo da Vinci (1452–1519) was a great painter, sculptor, architect and engineer. He believed that part of the job of an artist was to show things as they were, as exactly as possible.

Leonardo was very interested in anatomy. He felt that painters and sculptors could only show the human body properly if they understood how it was put together. Leonardo dissected about 30 bodies and made many notes and drawings.

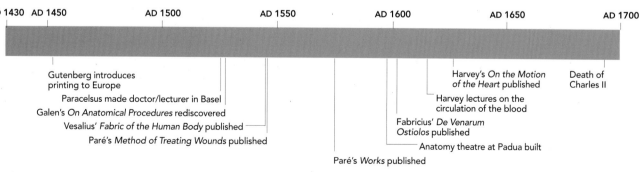

▲ **Early Modern medicine 1430–1700.**

A new book on anatomy by Galen

By the time of the Middle Ages most of Galen's books had been lost. Doctors only had bits and pieces of his books about anatomy. These had been translated from Arabic. After 1500 doctors wanted to know more. So Galen's books were translated and printed for all doctors to read. In 1531 Galen's most important book on anatomy was printed. It was called *On Anatomical Procedures*. This book had been lost in Europe since the fall of the Roman Empire. Doctors were delighted. Here was a book that said you must start with the skeleton. You must look carefully at the human body.

Vesalius

Vesalius was born into a medicial family in Brussels in 1514. He studied medicine at home, at Louvain and in Paris. He was fascinated by human dissection (which was allowed). But he really wanted to boil up a human body and get a skeleton (not allowed).

How Vesalius got a skeleton

Vesalius went to a gibbet outside the town of Louvain. On the gibbet was a dried up body of a criminal. All the flesh had gone. The bones were held together by the ligaments.

'I climbed the stake and pulled off the femur from the hip bone. The shoulder blades together with the arms and hands followed, although the fingers of one hand, both knee caps and one foot were missing.

Later I allowed myself to be shut out of the city in the evening in order to obtain the trunk, which was firmly held by a chain. The next day I transported the bones home through another gate in the city.'

Source C

As poles to tents, and walls to houses, so are bones to living creatures.

▲ From *On Anatomical Procedures*, written by Galen in about AD 200, lost until 1531.

Source D

I would let him cut me as often as he has cut man or other animal [except when eating].

▲ Vesalius on Johannes Guinter. He means Guinter had done little surgery or dissection.

Source E

I yield to none in my devotion and reverence to Galen.

▲ Vesalius, answering to criticism that he was against Galen.

Vesalius at Padua

In 1537 Vesalius went to Padua in Italy. He taught surgery and anatomy.

Teaching anatomy

Vesalius taught anatomy by doing his own dissections. This was a change because teachers had usually let an assistant do them. Vesalius made another change too. He published drawings of his dissections. He said these drawings would help students to understand what they were seeing during a dissection lesson.

The Tabulae Sex

In 1538 Vesalius published the *Tabulae Sex*. It was made up of six large sheets of drawings. In some of the drawings Vesalius shows the human liver just as Galen described it – with five lobes. But Galen had not been allowed to cut up humans, only animals. In fact animals have five lobed livers, humans only have two lobes. One of Vesalius' drawings shows a two lobed liver. Vesalius was beginning to question what Galen said.

Venesection

Venesection is the bleeding of sick people. Some doctors said only a small amount of blood should be taken. It should be taken on the opposite side of the body from the side that was sick. However, Vesalius wanted to get back to the ideas of Hippocrates and Galen who suggested taking more blood. Also, they had not said anything about which side of the body to take it from. Vesalius did drawings of the veins and gave reasons why the ideas of Hippocrates and Galen were right.

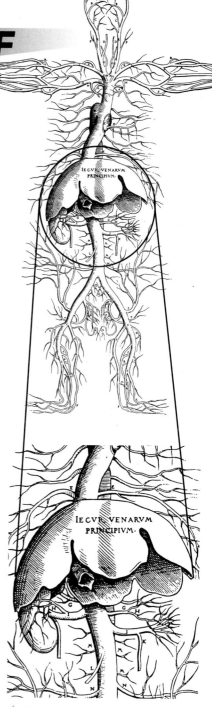

Source **F**

▲ A picture from the *Tabulae Sex*, by Vesalius published in 1538. It shows the ideas of Galen. The liver (see detail) is shown as a five lobed organ as Galen described it. This is the shape of an animal liver, not a human liver, which has only two lobes.

The Fabric of the Human Body 1543

This was Vesalius' great book on anatomy. The drawings were by first class artists. The publication of this book was an important moment in the history of medicine. Here are some of the reasons why it was so important.

Why *The Fabric of the Human Body* was important

1 The pictures were drawn from real human bodies.
2 Vesalius starts with the outside and works in. The part on the muscles starts with a picture of a body with the skin removed. This shows the surface muscles. Each picture after that shows deeper and deeper muscles.
3 Vesalius corrected some of Galen's mistakes in anatomy.
4 It was a new way of teaching – public dissection backed up with pictures.
5 It was a new type of book. Vesalius used the pictures to tell the story.
6 Vesalius spent months making sure all the wood blocks that were cut to print the pictures were absolutely correct to the smallest detail.
7 Vesalius' book was printed (not hand written) so there were lots of copies. Soon every medical school in Europe had a copy of *The Fabric of the Human Body*.

Vesalius' later life

Although at the time some old fashioned doctors disagreed with him, Vesalius' ideas changed the way anatomy was taught. His work was based on human dissection and, therefore, hard to argue with.

Vesalius wrote other books and became a doctor at the court of the Emperor, Charles V. He left the court in 1564 to go back to teaching in Padua but he died before he arrived there.

Source G

▲ The 16th picture from Vesalius' description of the muscles. Notice the letters and numbers which link the pictures to Vesalius' words.

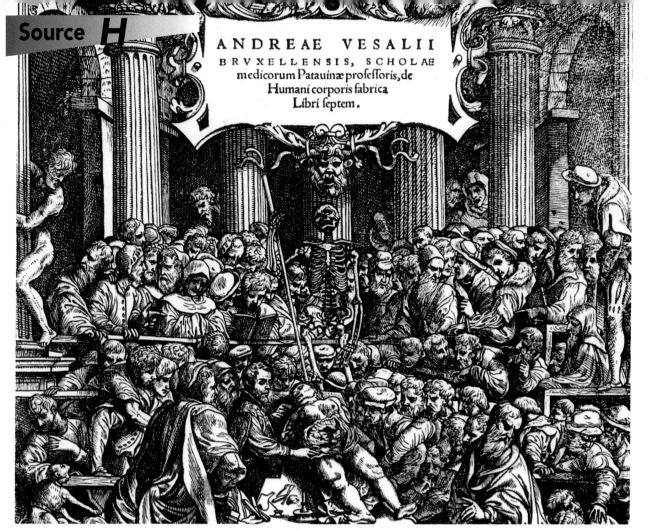

ANDREAE VESALII
BRVXELLENSIS, SCHOLAE
medicorum Patauinæ profeſſoris, de
Humani corporis fabrica
Libri ſeptem.

▲ The front page of *The Fabric of the Human Body*. Vesalius is doing the dissection outside. This was common at the time. Wooden stands were built so as many people as possible could watch.

TRENDS AND TURNING POINTS

A **trend** is a gradual change. It is made up of a series of events.

A **turning point** is a quick change. It may be just one event. Afterwards, things are never the same.

JOHANNES OPORINUS

Johannes Oporinus (1507–68) was the son of an artist in Basel. He worked as a manuscript copier, and also checked printed manuscripts.

Oporinus became interested in medicine. He went to Basel University to study medicine and studied under Paracelsus (see page 61). He did not get on with Paracelsus. He gave up studying medicine. He began to work as a lecturer in Latin and Greek at the university instead.

By 1536 Oporinus was a partner in a printing firm. The firm collapsed. In 1539 he started a new printing business, on his own. Vesalius probably chose Oporinus as his printer because he had such a wide range of knowledge and experience. He had medical training. He could speak Greek, Latin and Hebrew (all of these were used in the book). He spent a lot of time and money on *The Fabric of the Human Body*. He spent so much on it that the book had to be sold at a loss!

9.3 Ambroise Paré

Barber-surgeons

Ambroise Paré was the son of a barber-surgeon. Barber-surgeons were looked down on by doctors.

To Paris and the army

Paré went to Paris to train as a barber-surgeon in 1523. Although he became a good surgeon he does not seem to have had the money to take the examinations. He joined the French army. Since France was often at war, he became an expert in gunshot wounds. In 1545 he wrote a book about how to treat gunshot wounds.

Surgeon to the king

In 1552 Paré became surgeon to the king of France. He wrote more books. But the Faculty of Physicians attacked him. They said he was ignorant. (He was only a barber-surgeon.) And they said that the Faculty had to approve all books published. However, the king was on Paré's side so his books carried on selling.

The *Apology and Treatise of Ambroise Paré* – 1585

In 1585 Paré wrote his own life story. It was called the *Apology and Treatise of Ambroise Paré*. He wrote about the cases he had treated. He also wrote to explain the way he worked. Sources J, K and L are from Paré's book.

Source I

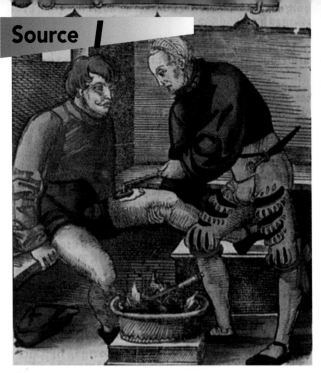

▲ This picture shows the old treatment of gunshot wounds. Gunshot wounds were thought to be poisonous. They were treated by burning with a red hot iron (cautery) or they were filled with boiling oil.

Source J

Dare you say you will teach me surgery, you who have never come out of your study? Surgery is learned by the eye and the hands. I can perform surgical operations which you cannot do, because you have never left your study or the schools. Diseases are not to be cured by talking. You do nothing else but chatter in a chair.

[Later Paré describes a battlefield covered with many dead men and horses]. So many blue and green flies rose from them they hid the sun; where they settled they infested the air and brought the plague with them.

▲ From the *Apology and Treatise of Ambroise Paré*, 1585. He is writing about a lecturer who criticized his work.

Source K

I had read that wounds made with weapons of fire were poisoned. They should be treated by cauterizing them with oil scalding hot mixed with a little treacle. Knowing it would cause great pain, I wanted to know what other surgeons did. They put on the oil as hot as possible. I took courage to do as they did.

Eventually I ran out of oil. I was forced to use an ointment made from yolks of eggs, oil of roses and turpentine.

That night I could not sleep. I was afraid what would happen because the wounds had not had burning oil. I rose early. To my surprise I found those to whom I gave my ointment feeling little pain and their wounds without inflammation or swelling. Whereas the others, on whom I used boiling oil, were feverish, with great pain and swelling about the edges of the wound.

Then I decided with myself never so cruelly to burn poor men wounded with gunshot.

▲ The story of how Paré discovered a new treatment for gunshot wounds.

Source L

Amputation
Let us suppose that a foot needs to be amputated. Let the patient be fed with meats, yolks of eggs, and bread toasted and dipped in wine to [keep him strong].

Place the patient as fit. Draw the muscles back and tie with a ligature....When you have made your ligature cut the flesh to the bone with a sharp well-cutting knife or with a crooked knife.

When you come to the bone cut it with a little saw. Then you must smooth the edge of the bone that the saw has made rough.

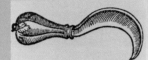 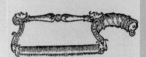

Bleeding
Let it bleed a little, then tie up the veins and arteries so that the course of the flowing blood may be stopped. This may be done by taking hold of the vessels with your Crow's Beak, which looks like this:

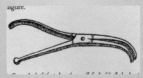

I used to stop the bleeding another way, of which I am ashamed, but what should I do? I had observed my masters who used hot irons. This kind of treatment could not but bring great pain to the patient. And truly of those that were burnt, only about a third of them recovered. I entreat all surgeons to leave this old and too cruel way and embrace this new.

▲ From *Of Amputations*, which appeared in Paré's *Works*, 1575.

Some years ago a certain gentleman had a bezoar stone. These stones were thought to be an antidote [cure] for all poisons. He bragged about it to King Charles. The king asked me whether there could be an antidote for all poisons. I said no because all poisons were different. I also said that it was an easy matter to test the stone on someone condemned to be hanged. The idea pleased the king.

There was a cook who was to be hanged for stealing two silver dishes. The king asked the cook whether he would take the poison and then the antidote. He could then go free. The cook cheerfully agreed.

So he was given poison and then some bezoar. After a while he began to vomit and move his bowels, and to cry out that his inward parts were burnt with fire.

After an hour I went to him. He was on the ground like a beast, with his tongue thrust forth out of his mouth, his eyes fiery, with cold sweats, and blood flowing from his ears, nose, mouth, anus and penis. At length he died in great torment seven hours after he took the poison.

▲ From *Of Bezoar* part of Paré's *Works*, 1575.

The importance of Paré

Paré was important for two reasons.

1 Paré understood how to test out a theory to see whether it was worth following or not (see Source M). This is at the heart of modern scientific thinking.

2 Paré also wanted to make all his new ideas public. This was so that other doctors could learn from him. The only way that medicine could progress was if doctors learnt from each other.

QUESTIONS

1 Read the caption to Source I on page 66. How were gunshot wounds treated before Paré?

2 Read Source K on page 67.

   a What was Paré's ointment for gunshot wounds made of?

   b What part did **chance** play in Paré's discovery of a new treatment for gunshot wounds? Choose the best sentence from the ones below.

   He thought boiling oil did not work.

   He ran out of boiling oil.

   He hated causing pain.

3 Read **Bleeding** in Source L on page 67.

   a How did surgeons stop bleeding before Paré?

   b How did Paré stop bleeding?

4 Read **The importance of Paré**. Give two reasons why Paré is important in the history of medicine.

Your brain tells you what you see

Is the drawing on the right a vase or the black shapes of two people facing each other? You can see it both ways. This is because our brain decides what we see. This is one of the reasons why doctors dissecting the human body did not immediately see how it worked. They had been taught to see the body through Galen's system, so they saw the things Galen's system made them expect to see.

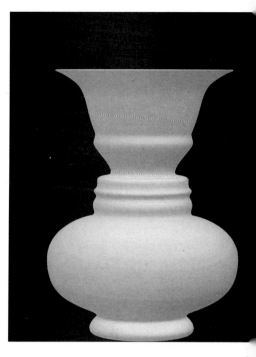

Things you already know

Things you already know help you to understand the world around you. Galen lived in Roman times. He knew about fire, metal smelting and brewing. He used ideas of these things when he thought about how the body worked. William Harvey grew up in a time when pumps were beginning to be used. There were pumps to pump water out of mines. There were also pumps to pump water to put out fires. When Harvey thought about how the heart worked, he could compare it to a pump because he had seen pumps working. Galen had not.

Vesalius changes his mind

At first Vesalius accepted Galen's idea that blood passed from one side of the heart to the other through the septum. Later he disagreed. He said there were definitely no holes. The blood could not pass through the septum.

Realdo Colombo and Geronimo Fabricius

Realdo Colombo worked at Padua after Vesalius. He showed that blood passed from one side of the heart to the other via the lungs. Geronimo Fabricius, another professor of anatomy at Padua, noticed the valves in the veins (1603). Fabricius taught William Harvey who was later to become very famous.

Source N

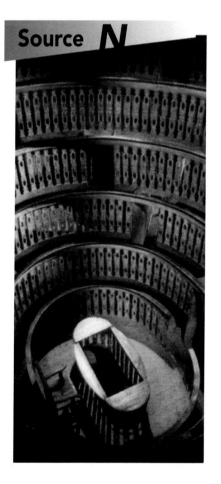

▶ The anatomy theatre at Padua, built by Fabricius in 1594. Everyone could see what was going on.

William Harvey

Harvey was born in 1578 and studied medicine at Padua. Afterwards he worked in London as a doctor and a teacher of anatomy. He was doctor to James I and Charles I.

Harvey and live hearts

Harvey wanted to find out how the heart worked. He needed live hearts. He worked on animals, but most of them had such fast heartbeats he could not see what was happening. He then worked on frogs because they have a slow heartbeat.

Pumping blood

Harvey saw that each time the heart contracted (went smaller) it pumped out a lot of blood. He worked out how much blood the heart was pumping out. He decided that there was too much blood for it all to be used up, and for the body to make new blood all the time (as Galen said).

Harvey and the circulation of blood

Harvey said there must be a fixed amount of blood in the body. All the blood **circulated** (moved around) the body. It was pumped round by the heart.

Harvey and the valves in veins

Harvey worked out an experiment to show that the little flaps or valves in the veins only allowed blood to flow one way. Now he could show that the blood flowed out from the heart through the arteries. It flowed back through the veins.

Harvey's book about the heart

Harvey published *An Anatomical Treatise on the Motion of the Heart* in 1628. This put forward all his ideas about the blood circulating.

Source O

The two movements of the heart happen so quickly they cannot be seen separately.

It seems to be a single movement. This is like when you pull the trigger of a gun, a flint strikes steel. A spark happens and lights the powder. The flame spreads. The bullet flies out. All these movements happen so quickly you cannot see them separately.

▲ From *An Anatomical Treatise on the Motion of the Heart*, written by William Harvey in 1628.

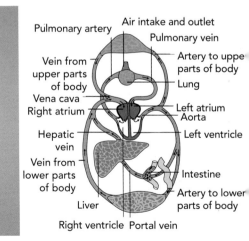

▲ Harvey's physiological system.

Source P

The pump has two valves. One to open when the handle is lifted up and when it is down to shut. The other is to open to let the water out. At the end of the machine a man holds a copper pipe turning it from side to side to where the fire shall be.

▲ Salomon de Caus describing a machine for putting out fires, 1615.

Source Q

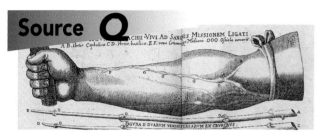

▲ An illustration from Fabricius' book showing the valves in the veins.

Source R

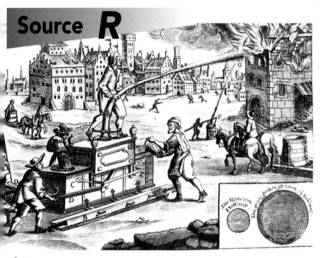

▲ A pump for putting out fires, 1673.

Source S

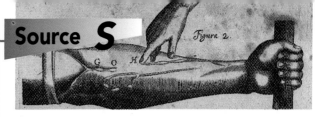

▲ From Harvey's book, 1628. It shows how valves in the veins allow blood to flow in just one direction.

WILLIAM HARVEY

William Harvey (1578–1657) became a doctor at the age of 24 (see page 70). He returned to England from Padua (where he had studied) in 1602.

In 1607 Harvey joined the Royal College of Surgeons and also became the chief physician at St Bartholomew's Hospital (which cared for the poor). He had to promise not to charge the patients for his work. He also had to go to the hospital at least once a week. Harvey also had his own medical practice. He did charge his private patients for looking after them.

In 1615 Harvey became a lecturer in anatomy at the Royal College of Surgeons. He did not give up his private practice (he even became doctor to the royal family). He did give up his work at St Bartholomew's.

During the English Civil War Harvey was a Royalist. He did not actually fight, but travelled with the royal family as their doctor. He carried on dissecting bodies and making experiments as they all moved around the country.

When the war ended, Harvey returned to live in London. He opened his private medical practice again. He started lecturing and experimenting. He died of gout.

9.5 Treatment

New Ideas

There were many new ideas in medicine and anatomy in the Early Modern period. Vesalius and Harvey discovered a great deal about how the body worked. Their ideas were more scientific. They were based on close observation.

New treatment?

But there was very little new treatment in the Early Modern period. Paré knew that some things worked but he did not know why. The next two pages show some of the treatments used in the 1600s.

THE DOCTOR – THOMAS SYDENHAM

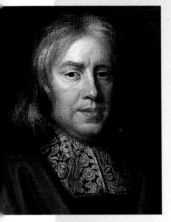

Sydenham was one of the most successful doctors in London from 1656 to his death in 1689. Here is his advice to a young man who wanted to be a doctor.

'Anatomy, botany – nonsense. Sir, I know an old woman in the flower market who understands botany better. As for anatomy, my butcher can dissect a joint just as well. No young man. You must go to the bedside. It is there alone you can learn about disease.'

Sydenham often thought the best treatment was to leave the patient alone. Other treatments were based on common sense. Roast chicken and a bottle of wine was his treatment for a man weakened by too many bleedings and purgings.

Because of his close observation by the bedside [like Hippocrates] he discovered the disease of **scarlet fever**.

In a letter to another doctor Sydenham said:

'I have been careful to write only what was the result of faithful observation.'

WOMEN

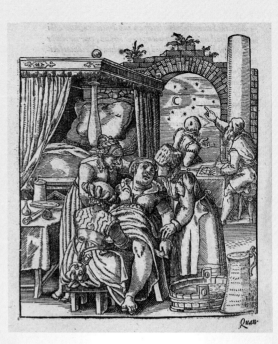

Women as midwives
This picture comes from a book printed in 1580. It shows a woman giving birth. But things had not changed by the 17th century. The woman is being helped by a midwife and comforted by friends. The two doctors are casting the baby's horoscope. Midwives were usually women. Sometimes they had trained with another midwife.

Women surgeons and doctors
There were a few women surgeons and doctors in 17th century England. But they were less common than in the Middle Ages. Men took over medicine.

Nursing
There were some nurses but mostly a sick person was nursed by his or her family.

Healers
Many sick people did not go to a qualified doctor. They could not afford to or they did not want to. Some went to healers who might be wise women or wizards, or even the lady of the manor. If you were sick in the 1600s you might have been more likely to see a woman healer than a male doctor.

DIFFERENT TYPES OF TREATMENT

If you are ill today you will probably see a doctor working in western medicine. But there are other treatments: acupuncture, faith healing and homoeopathy are all types of healing used in Britain today.

There were even more different treatments in Britain in the 17th century.

When we read letters and diaries written by people at the time, we see they used many different treatments. They used supernatural cures as well as herbs and medicines. Even doctors used different cures. Sometimes they used supernatural cures.

Robert Burton was a doctor. He warned against supernatural cures because they often worked! He thought that this was the work of the Devil:

'Evil should not be done even if good come of it. Much better for such patients to suffer misery rather than risk their soul forever. It is better that they die rather than be cured this way.'

LADY MARGARET HOBY

Lady Margaret Hoby (1571–1633) lived at a time when many rich women knew some herbal cures. They were expected to care for their families and the people on the land their families owned.

Lady Margaret saw most of her patients at her home. She gave herbal cures and cleaned and bandaged wounds.

Lady Margaret was unusual because she did not just use herbal cures. She tried all sorts of other cures, including minor surgery. She also set broken bones.

CHARLES II

In 1685 Charles II was dying. He had the best doctors in England. Even so, his treatment sounds terrible.

One of his doctors, Sir Charles Scarburgh, wrote a description of the treatment:

2 February *The king felt some unusual disturbance in his brain, soon followed by loss of speech and fits. Two of the king's doctors opened a vein in his right arm, and drew off about 16 ounces [454 grams] of blood.*

The treatment continued:

Eight more ounces [227 grams] of blood let, then pills to 'drain away the humours', and medicine to make him vomit.

3 February *Sacred Tincture every six hours [a laxative]. Ten ounces [280 grams] of blood let from the jugular veins, after which the king said he had a sore throat.*

4 February *More laxative. Then, as Charles got worse, a medicine which included 40 drops of essence of human skull.*

5 February *Peruvian bark [quinine].*

6 February *His Majesty's strength was failing. A heart tonic was tried, then a medicine including Bezoar Stone.*

Charles died.

One of the best ways of finding out about the attitudes of ordinary people to medicine is to read their diaries. The most comprehensive of these is the diary left by Samuel Pepys which covers the years 1660–69. Pepys was a civil servant working for the navy in the 1660s. Pepys' diary is famous for its coverage of the plague of 1665 and the Fire of London in 1660. But it also discusses Pepys' daily life in great detail, including his ailments and those of his wife, both major and minor.

The entries show us how common minor infections were at the time, and how hard they were to get rid of without antibiotics. They also show us that people were prepared to shop around for advice, consulting a variety of doctors and apothecaries. It is also clear that it was perfectly acceptable for someone like Pepys to just wander in and watch operations and experiments.

18 January 1661: I took Mr Hollier [a surgeon who had operated on Pepys for bladder stone] to the Greyhound – where he did advise me above all things to avoid drinking often; which I am resolved if I can to leave off.

26 February 1663: To Surgeons' Hall where we were led into the [Anatomy] Theatre. Dr Tearne began his lecture upon the kidneys, ureter and penis, which was very fine. After dinner Dr Scarburgh took some of his friends, and I went along with them, to see the body alone: which we did. I did touch the dead body with my bare hand; it felt cold but methought it was a very unpleasant sight. Thence we went into a private room where they prepare the bodies, and there was the kidneys etc. on which he had lectured today. And Dr Scarburgh did show very clearly the manner of the disease of the Stone, and the cutting, and all other questions I can think of. And so to the afternoon lecture upon the heart, lungs etc.

1 July 1664: By and by comes Dr Burnett – who assures me I have an ulcer either in the Kidneys or Bladder; for my urine, which he saw yesterday, he is sure the sediment is not slime gathered by heat, but direct pus. He did write me down some directions what to do for it. It is strange Mr Hollier should never say one word of this ulcer in all his life to me.

Dr Burnett's prescription and advice
...Dissolve one spoonful of this syrup in every glass of ale or beer you drink. Morning and evening swallow the quantity of a hazelnut of Cyprus Turpentine. If you are constipated or suffer a fit of the Stone eat an ounce of Cassia [a cheap type of cinnamon] newly drawn, from the point of a knife.

Old Canary and Malaga wine you may drink to three or four glasses, but no new wine, and what wine you drink, let it be at meals.

CHAPTER 10

MEDICINE ON THE BRINK

10.1 The old order begins to change

New discoveries in science

The interest in science continued in the 18th century. Some new discoveries were made. These included:

- The microscope (1683)
- The thermometer (1709 by Fahrenheit and 1742 by Celsius)
- Gases, such as hydrogen and oxygen.

Medicine

The new discoveries in science did not change anything in medicine for some time. Even so, medicine did not stand still.

Hermann Boerhaave was a doctor who told his students to watch patients carefully and take notes (see box).

Other doctors studied breathing and digestion.

Surgery improved and operations were faster. William Cheselden could take a stone out of the bladder in one minute!

Patients were glad of such speed, as there were no effective anaesthetics at this time!

HERMANN BOERHAAVE

Hermann Boerhaave taught medicine in Holland between 1718 and 1729. He taught his students to take careful notes, to make use of new ideas in science, and to do post mortems so they could work out why someone had died. His students spread his ideas all over the world. One of them, Alexander Monro, turned Edinburgh University into a great medical centre.

JOHN HUNTER

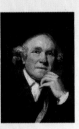

John Hunter (1728–93) is often called the 'Father of Modern Surgery'. He started his studies by doing dissections for his famous brother, William. John became a surgeon and invented new operations such as **tracheotomy** (to clear air passages). He built up a collection of anatomical specimens [bones and organs from people and animals] for doctors to study.

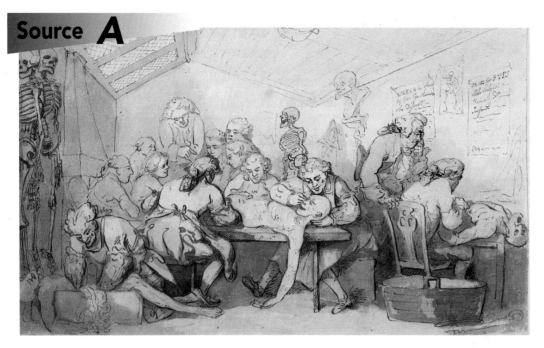

◀A drawing of William Hunter's dissecting room towards the end of the 18th century.

Respect for doctors?

Surgeons became more respected during the 18th century. The Royal College of Surgeons was founded in 1800. People came to think that sick people should be properly looked after. Rich people began to set up hospitals.

Old ideas

However, many doctors still used old fashioned ideas. They used the ideas of the four humours. They thought disease could be spread by **miasmas** (bad air).

Quackery

There were, and always had been, quack doctors. They sold useless pills or sugared water that they said would cure everything.

New ideas

A German doctor, Franz Mesmer (1734–1815), used hypnotism to treat patients.

▶ **Doctors sniffing the gold tops of their walking sticks which contain a liquid they thought prevented them from catching disease.**

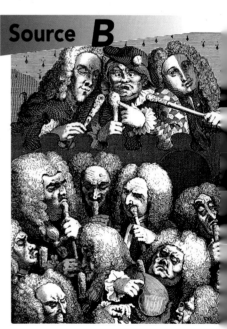

THE IRISH GIANT

John O'Brien was almost 2.5m tall. His friends sold his body to the anatomist John Hunter for £500. O'Brien had asked them not to let Hunter have his body. Hunter put the skeleton in his anatomy museum.

10.2 The situation in 1820

The state of medicine in 1820

1 Doctors still did not know what really caused disease.

2 Doctors did not know much about chemistry.

3 Doctors only had simple microscopes. They had no complicated machines to help them.

4 Surgeons did not know about infection. They did not wash before operating on people.

5 There were no proper anaesthetics. People often died from the shock of the pain.

6 During operations people often lost a lot of blood. **Blood transfusions** did not work because no one knew about blood groups.

THE GROWTH OF INDUSTRY

First Phase – 1780–1875
- **1781** The steam engine was perfected. Steam engines powered everything from pumps in coal mines to railway engines and machines to spin cotton.

- **1840s** Railways meant that people, goods and letters travelled quicker than ever before.

- **1850–75** Britain became rich by selling goods all over the world.

Second Phase – 1875–1900
- The USA, Germany and France caught up with Britain.
- New industries grew up: motor cars, firms making chemicals, firms making electrical goods like light bulbs and cookers.
- New materials came into use, including steel, rubber and aluminium.

Third Phase – 1900 onwards
- The age of high technology. Many new machines were invented. These included machines to help doctors: kidney dialysis machines (1945) and body scanners (1970s).

10.3 The impact of the Industrial Revolution

Starting in the late 18th century many changes took place in Britain. These changes are often called the **Industrial Revolution**.

1 The population grew.

2 More people wanted goods. Factories were started up to produce these goods.

3 At first the new factories were powered by water. Then they were powered by steam. Much later they were powered by electricity.

4 Many more people moved to the towns to work. Towns grew, but most of the new houses were badly built. There was more disease.

5 But scientists made new discoveries. This helped to conquer disease. For example, a better microscope was invented. This helped doctors to discover germs.

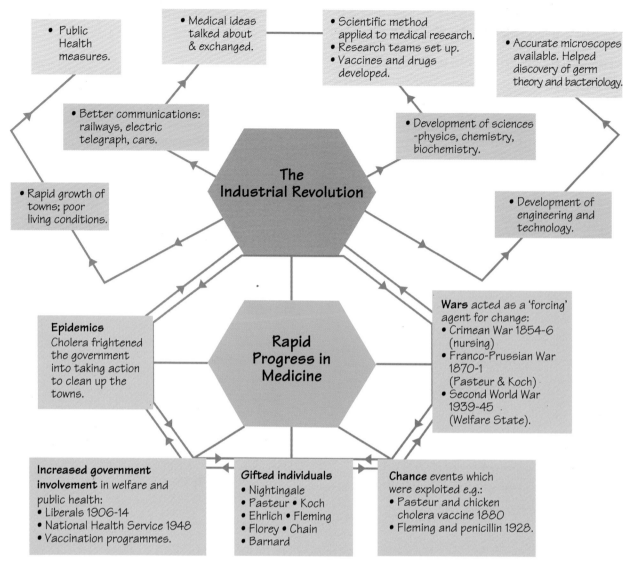

The web of factors which enabled medicine to progress very quickly after about 1850.

Content of diagram:

- Public Health measures.
- Medical ideas talked about & exchanged.
- Scientific method applied to medical research.
- Research teams set up.
- Vaccines and drugs developed.
- Accurate microscopes available. Helped discovery of germ theory and bacteriology.
- Better communications: railways, electric telegraph, cars.
- Development of sciences -physics, chemistry, biochemistry.
- Rapid growth of towns; poor living conditions.
- Development of engineering and technology.

The Industrial Revolution

Rapid Progress in Medicine

Epidemics Cholera frightened the government into taking action to clean up the towns.

Wars acted as a 'forcing' agent for change:
- Crimean War 1854-6 (nursing)
- Franco-Prussian War 1870-1 (Pasteur & Koch)
- Second World War 1939-45 (Welfare State).

Increased government involvement in welfare and public health:
- Liberals 1906-14
- National Health Service 1948
- Vaccination programmes.

Gifted individuals
- Nightingale
- Pasteur • Koch
- Ehrlich • Fleming
- Florey • Chain
- Barnard

Chance events which were exploited e.g.:
- Pasteur and chicken cholera vaccine 1880
- Fleming and penicillin 1928.

The medical revolution – 1850-the present day

Look at the diagram above. This shows all the things that helped to make medicine progress very quickly from about 1850 to the present day. This was far faster than medicine had progressed in the 3000 years before. This rapid progress is often called the **medical revolution**.

PINEL

Until the 18th century the mentally ill were often shut away in asylums. They were often chained up. Ordinary people visited these places as if they were zoos. In 1792 Philippe Pinel began to study madness. His asylum (in France) treated people more kindly.

CHAPTER 11

THE FIGHT AGAINST INFECTIOUS DISEASE

11.1 Edward Jenner and smallpox

Smallpox was a deadly disease. It killed a lot of people. Victims got a high fever and sores full of pus all over the body. Many died. Those who survived had terrible scars and were often blind. Some people tried inoculation but it did not always work (see box).

Edward Jenner (1749–1823)

Jenner was a doctor from Berkeley in Gloucestershire. He had studied with John Hunter, the famous surgeon.

Jenner had heard that milkmaids who had caught the mild disease, cowpox, did not catch smallpox. He studied the milkmaids in his area. Each time there was a smallpox epidemic, milkmaids who had had cowpox did not catch smallpox.

In 1796 Jenner gave a healthy boy cowpox. The boy got better. Jenner then deliberately gave him a dose of smallpox (see Source A). The boy did not fall ill! Jenner called this new method **vaccination**, after the Latin word *vacca* which means 'a cow'.

Jenner could not explain how vaccination worked. So work based on it was slow to follow.

INOCULATION

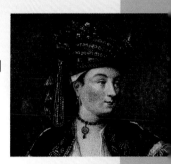

An English woman, Lady Mary Wortley Montagu, learned about inoculation in Turkey. She brought the idea to England in 1718. The patient's arm was cut. A thread soaked in pus from the sores of a victim who had a mild form of smallpox was pulled through the cut. Sometimes the patient had a mild dose of smallpox, then got better. They were then safe from the deadly form of smallpox. But sometimes the inoculation gave people a heavy dose of smallpox. These people died.

Source A

I chose James Phipps, a healthy boy about eight years old. The cowpox matter was put into his arm on 14 May 1796. A week later he was a little unwell but was soon fit. Then he was inoculated with smallpox but no disease followed.

▲ Adapted from the writings of Edward Jenner, 1798.

What other doctors thought

Many doctors did not support vaccination. Some of these doctors had been inoculating people for years and had made a lot of money.

Support for vaccination

However, lots of people supported vaccination. In other countries vaccination quickly became popular. Then in Britain some members of the royal family were vaccinated. This made it popular. Parliament even gave money to Jenner for his work. By 1853, vaccination was compulsory. This was surprising, because the government usually did not make laws about what people should do for the good of their health. Smallpox slowly began to disappear.

▼ A cartoon drawn by James Gillray in 1802 showing that some people were afraid of what vaccination would do.

Source C

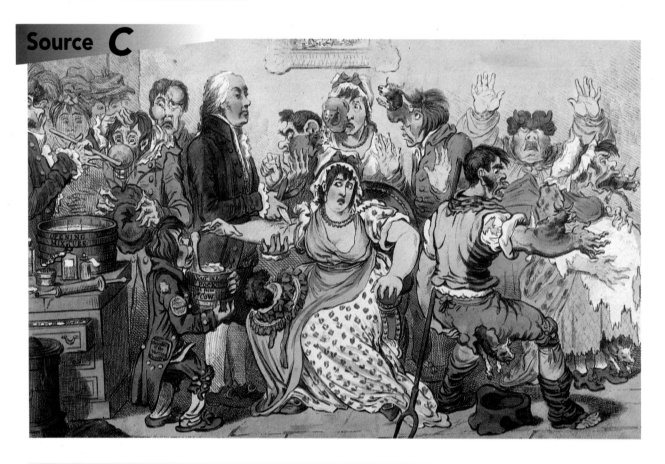

Source D

In 1799 John Ring met Edward Jenner. Then in 1808 Ring went to Ringwood in Hampshire to investigate some vaccination cases that were supposed to have failed. Feelings ran so high that he and his group had to carry pistols. When the British Vaccine Establishment was opened in 1809, Ring was the main vaccinator.

▲ From *The History of Wincanton* by George Sweetman, 1903.

Source E

After being vaccinated with cowpox she was very ill. Many years later she caught smallpox.

▲ C. Cooke, an apothecary, writing about a case in 1799.

Source F

In this publication it is noticed that there was a Parliamentary grant of £30,000 given to Dr Jenner for an unsuccessful experiment.

There is also a letter about the new and fatal disease, 'vaccine ulcer'. There is a letter from Ringwood proving the failures of vaccination there and a list of those who died of cowpox there.

▲ Public opposition to Jenner and smallpox vaccination in the press.

Source G

Medicine has never before made such a useful improvement. In the future, people will only know about smallpox through learning history.

▲ A letter to Jenner from the President of the USA, 1802.

JESTY

Benjamin Jesty was a famer in Dorset. He claimed that he had vaccinated his family against smallpox with cowpox in 1774. This was well before Jenner published the story of his vaccination of James Phipps in 1789.

Jesty was just one of several people to make this claim after Jenner's discovery was published. Jenner, not surprisingly, did not believe the claims. Jesty's claim was put forward by someone who was trying to discredit Jenner, so it looked even more like a fake. No matter who first used vaccination, it was Jenner who first made the discovery public.

SUMMARY

▶ Smallpox was a deadly epidemic disease in the 18th century.

▶ A English woman brought inoculation to Britain. But it was risky and did not stop many deaths from smallpox.

▶ Jenner saw that cowpox victims did not catch smallpox.

▶ Jenner vaccinated people with cowpox.

▶ Vaccination worked. So more and more people used it.

▶ Jenner could not explain how vaccination worked. So his work did not lead on to other discoveries.

Microscopes

Microscopes meant that scientists could see micro-organisms (germs). Could this get them nearer knowing what caused disease?

Ideas about disease in 1800

Some people believed in spontaneous generation. This theory said that germs were made by disease. They did not cause it. Some of these people believed that disease was caused by gases in the air called **miasmas**. Others had different ideas.

Pasteur and germs

Louis Pasteur was the scientist who made the first links between germs and disease. He was not looking for this link. He made his discoveries while trying to solve problems for various manufacturing businesses.

Germs and decay

First, Pasteur showed that germs caused things to **decay** (go bad). He did this when he was asked to find out what made alcohol go bad while it was fermenting. He heated water in a swan-neck flask. This drove the air around the bend in the neck. The air could not get back. But when the neck of the flask was broken the air and germs got in. Decay set in. So the germs must be in the air and cause decay.

LOUIS PASTEUR
(1822–95)

Louis Pasteur was a French chemist. He was the first person to make the connection between germs and disease.

In 1857 he investigated the problem of alcohol going bad and linked germs to decay.

In 1865 he began to investigate silkworm disease. His work was interrupted by the deaths of his father and two daughters.

In 1868 he had a brain haemorrhage and was paralysed on one side. By 1877 he was back at work.

Pasteur's achievements

- discovered that heating liquid kills germs. This is called 'pasteurization'.
- developed a vaccine for chicken cholera (1880).
- developed a vaccine for anthrax (1881).
- developed a vaccine for rabies (1885).

Source H

I boil some liquid in a long-necked flask. I let it cool. In a few days little animals will grow in it. But by boiling it I had killed the germs. If I repeat the experiment but draw the neck into a curve, but still open, the liquid will remain pure for three or four years. They both contain the same liquid and they both contain air. But the difference is that in one the dust in the air and its germs can fall in, in the other they cannot.

▲ Pasteur's description of the experiment he carried out in public at the University of Paris on 7 April 1864.

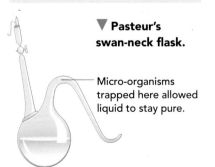

▼ Pasteur's swan-neck flask.

Micro-organisms trapped here allowed liquid to stay pure.

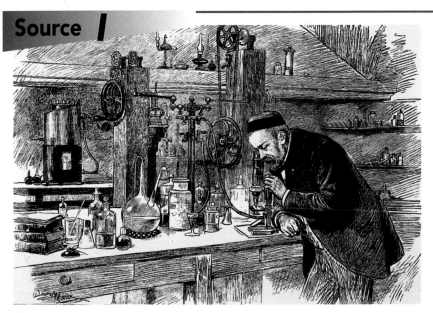

▲ This print of Pasteur working in his laboratory was made when Pasteur was famous.

11.3 Robert Koch

Pasteur proved that germs cause disease. He could not prove which germ caused which disease. It was a German doctor, Robert Koch, who did this.

Koch and anthrax

In 1872 Koch began to study **anthrax**, an animal disease that could spread to humans. He studied the blood of animals with and without the disease. By 1875 he had found the germ.

Koch and blood poisoning

Koch then studied the germ that caused blood poisoning. The germ was so small that he could not see it. How could he study it? How could he show it caused disease?

New technology

Koch used new chemical **dyes** to stain the germ so it could be seen. He then used a new kind of photographic lens to record how, under the microscope, the germ bred until it was the only germ in the blood. If it was the only germ then it must be the cause of the disease.

ROBERT KOCH
(1843–1910)

Robert Koch was a German doctor who first showed that a particular germ caused a particular disease.

Using the new discoveries in chemical dyes and photography, Koch could colour germs so they showed up clearly. He then photographed them.

In 1882 he discovered the germ that caused tuberculosis.

In 1883 he discovered the germ that caused cholera.

Koch won the Nobel Prize in 1905 for his work.

▼ Robert Koch is shown as St George defeating tuberculosis.

Source J

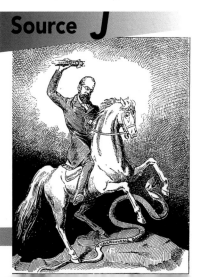

Germit hunters

Germ hunters

Soon everyone was looking for germs. Once the germs were discovered vaccines and drugs could be made.

Year	Microbe discovered	Name of scientist
1879	Leprosy	Hansen
1880	Typhoid	Eberth
1882	Diphtheria	Klebs
1884	Tetanus	Nicholaier
1884	Pneumonia	Frankael
1894	Plague	Kitasato and Yersin

PASTEUR'S TEAM

Many scientists worked with Pasteur. Charles Chamberland (left) helped discover how germs can be weakened. Emile Roux made discoveries about diphtheria. Alexander Yersin made discoveries about bubonic plague. Albert Calmette helped discover the vaccine for tuberculosis.

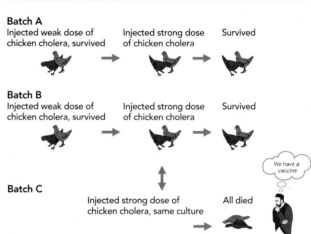

▲ How Pasteur discovered the principle of making vaccines from the germs of the chicken cholera disease.

11.4 Vaccines

Chicken cholera vaccine

Pasteur read about what Koch had discovered. He wanted to make more discoveries for France, because France had been beaten by Germany in the Franco-Prussian War of 1870–1. Pasteur built up a team of scientists to work with him. He was asked to look into the disease of chicken cholera.

Pasteur took some blood from sick chickens and grew the germs in a broth. His assistant, Charles Chamberland, was in charge of injecting the germ broth into the chickens. He went on holiday and left the broth in the flask, open to the air. When he got back he injected the chickens with the germ broth.

But they did not die. Chamberland told Pasteur what had happened. They made a new germ broth and injected the chickens again. But still they did not die (see Batch A above). They tried the whole thing all over again with a new batch of chickens. The chickens still did not die (Batch B). Finally, they injected another batch of chickens with a fresh broth of strong germs only. All of them died (Batch C).

Pasteur realized that leaving the broth uncovered had weakened the germs. The the weak germs had helped the chickens in Batches A and B to fight off the stronger, deadly germs. This way of making a vaccine is called **attenuation**.

Pasteur and anthrax

Pasteur wanted to find a vaccine for the deadly disease of anthrax. Dr. Emile Roux worked with Pasteur. Roux made a weak anthrax germ. Then came the test.

Testing the vaccine

In 1881 Pasteur was asked to prove that his new anthrax vaccine worked. He went to a farm near Paris. There were 60 sheep:

- 25 were injected with the weak anthrax germ (vaccine). Then later with a deadly dose of strong anthrax.
- 25 were injected with a deadly dose of strong anthrax.
- 10 were left alone.

Result

Within a month only the sheep that had been vaccinated were alive and well.

News of Pasteur's success was reported all over the world. Soon many animals were vaccinated against anthrax.

The death rate from anthrax in animals went down quickly. Farmers were saved a lot of money.

This research helped human medicine too. It made people happier about vaccination. If it worked on animals it would also work on humans.

Source K

Will you have some microbe? There is some everywhere. The learned Monsieur Pasteur, has spoken. The microbe alone is the characteristic of a disease.

▲ From an article in the *Veterinary Press* which made fun of the germ theory.

Source L

Paris 2 June. 9.30pm [by telegraph from our correspondents]
Today I went to see the result of an experiment by M. Pasteur.

On 5 May, 25 sheep were marked with a hole in their ear and injected with anthrax vaccine.

On 31 May all 50 sheep were injected with the anthrax vaccine.

By 2 June, 23 of the unvaccinated sheep were dead. Two more died an hour later. The sheep which had been vaccinated frolicked and stayed healthy.

▲ A report from *The Times*, Friday 3 June 1881.

PROFESSOR COLIN

Professor Colin believed in spontaneous generation (see page 82). He said Pasteur cheated at Pouilly-le-Fort. The germs had sunk to the bottom of the flask, then liquid from the top had been used. A quick shake of the flask proved him wrong.

Rabies

Rabies is a deadly disease. Pasteur wanted to make a rabies vaccine. His assistant, Emile Roux, kept the spines of dead rabbits who had died of rabies. He kept testing to see how long the rabies germ stayed alive in the dead spine.

Pasteur sees Roux's work

Pasteur copied Roux's idea. Roux was angry. Pasteur began to test a vaccine from the rabbit's spines on dogs. He injected a dog with weak germs from a 14 day-old rabbit spine. Then a 13 day-old spine and so on. The last injection contained very strong germs from the spine of a freshly dead rabbit. The dogs he treated like this did not get rabies.

The boy who was dying of rabies

Pasteur was not sure if the rabies vaccine would work on humans. Then one day in 1885, **Joseph Meister** arrived at Pasteur's laboratory. He was covered with bites from a rabid dog. He was going to die anyway. Pasteur decided to try injecting the vaccine. It worked. Soon Pasteur vaccinated lots of people against rabies.

Diphtheria

The germ of diphtheria was discovered by **Edwin Klebs**, a German doctor. But he could not find out how to stop the disease. Many scientists, including Emile Roux and **Emil von Behring** (a student of Robert Koch), worked to find an injection to prevent the disease.

Tuberculosis

Koch was working on a vaccine for tuberculosis (TB). The German government pressed him to show how good it was at an International Medical Congress in 1890. Lots of people with tuberculosis flocked to see Koch but the vaccine did not work. Koch was blamed but work on finding new vaccines went on.

Governments

The French government knew that the work of Pasteur made France famous. The German government felt the same way about Koch. Both men were given money and buildings where they could carry on their research.

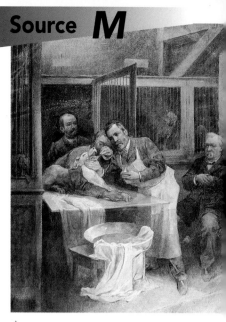

▲ Removing saliva from a rabid dog.

Joseph Meister, aged nine years, was knocked over and bitten by a rabid dog.

Some bites were so deep as to make walking difficult. The dog was certainly rabid.

The death of this child being certain, I decided to try the method which had been successful with dogs.

Meister was injected with liquid from the spine of a rabbit which had died of rabies fifteen days before.

He survived.

▲ Pasteur's description of the rabies injection.

Industry, science & technology

• The much improved microscope allowed bacteria to be studied.
• Koch used industrial chemical dyes to stain bacteria.

Communications

• The results of experiments and research were spread quickly via telegraph, newspapers and journals. Railways enabled scientists to meet regularly.

Research techniques

• Both Pasteur and Koch devised experiments to prove theories.
• Both had research teams.

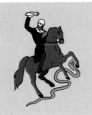

Factors which enabled Pasteur and Koch to succeed

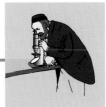

Personal qualities

• Both men were intelligent, persistent and determined.
• Both spoke in public at the risk of abuse from doubters.

Chance events

• Chamberland's 'mistake' when Pasteur was researching a vaccine for chicken cholera.
• The surprise arrival of Joseph Meister allowed Pasteur to test his rabies vaccine on humans.

War

• The Franco-Prussian War (1870–1) ended in a disastrous defeat for the French. Tension between the two countries followed.
• Pasteur and Koch were spurred on by this tension. They became rivals; a new discovery brought prestige for their country.

THOUILLER

Louis Thouiller was a young assistant in Louis Pasteur's research team. In 1883 he went with Roux to Egypt, where cholera had broken out. They went to study the cholera germ. So did a German research team, led by Koch.

Soon the French team announced that they had isolated the germ. But they had also been exposed to cholera. Thouiller caught the disease.

Koch tested the French results. They had made a mistake. They had confused platelets, a normal part of blood, for the germ. Thouiller knew that Koch was testing the French results. He asked Koch to visit him. When Koch arrived he asked if the results were right. Koch let the dying man believe that he had isolated the cholera germ. He did not make the mistake public until Thouiller was dead.

SUMMARY

▶ **1850** No one knew what caused disease.

▶ **1857** Pasteur discovered that something in the air caused sugar beet juice to go bad.

▶ **1864** Pasteur proved his germ theory [that germs are in the air] in a public experiment in Paris.

▶ Robert Koch started to study anthrax. He proved that one sort of germ caused one sort of disease.

▶ Pasteur and Koch built up teams of scientists to help them to make lmore discoveries.

▶ All the scientists learned from each other. The electric telegraph, railways and newspapers meant that scientists learnt what other scientists were doing.

An infectious disease is a disease you can catch from someone else. This includes colds, 'flu, chicken-pox and measles. In the past it included diphtheria, smallpox and cholera.

Keeping clean

Germs grow best in dirt. So governments passed laws to make sure sewage was taken away from houses and that clean water was piped into houses.

Vaccines

By 1900 scientists, like Pasteur, had discovered germs. They had made vaccines to prevent people and animals catching terrible diseases such as rabies and anthrax. They knew what caused infectious diseases and how to prevent healthy people from getting them.

But no one knew how to kill off the germs in a person who already had the disease (without killing the person as well).

Paul Ehrlich and the magic bullet

Paul Ehrlich first worked on diphtheria. He was fascinated to see the way that the body made **antibodies**.

These antibodies could attack and destroy germs in a person's body. The antibodies homed in on the germs like a **magic bullet**. Sometimes the antibodies did not succeed. They needed help.

Ehrlich wanted to find a **chemical** that homed in on a certain germ and killed that germ inside the sick person.

PAUL EHRLICH

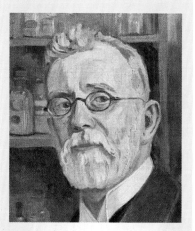

Ehrlich was born in Germany in 1854.

He studied chemistry and bacteriology [study of germs]. He worked as a doctor.

In 1889, after he had recovered from tuberculosis (TB), he joined Koch's team at the Institute for Infectious Diseases in Berlin.

He helped Behring in his research on diphtheria.

From 1899 he studied the treatment of disease with chemicals.

He shared the Nobel Prize for medicine in 1908.

He died in 1915.

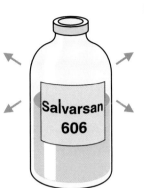

Industry

Progress in the chemical industry provided Ehrlich with the idea that chemicals (e.g. synthetic dyes) might be able to kill germs inside the body.

Personal Qualities

Ehrlich was determined and skilful. He was inspired by Koch and Behring.

Science and Technology

Improved knowledge of physics and skilled engineering provided Ehrlich with technical aids (e.g. the microscope).

Research Techniques

Teamwork and careful observation were crucial. Hata had the patience to re-check previous work.

◀ Factors involved in the discovery of Salvarsan 606.

The search for a chemical to destroy syphilis

Syphilis was a sexually transmitted disease that killed thousands of people every year. Ehrlich and his team made up and tested over 600 mixtures of arsenic. They hoped that one of them might kill the syphilis germ. All of them seemed to be useless.

Sahachiro Hata

Hata was Japanese. He joined Ehrlich's team in 1909. He was asked to re-test the arsenic mixtures that had been tested and rejected. To his surprise he found that mixture number 606 worked. It did kill the syphilis germ. Perhaps someone made a mistake before.

Salvarsan 606

Ehrlich called the new medicine, Salvarsan 606. He found it worked on rabbits with syphilis without killing the rabbits. Because it had arsenic (a poison) in it, he insisted on tests on hundreds of rabbits before it was tried on people. In 1911 it was tried on a human being. It worked.

Doctors against Salvarsan 606

Some doctors said Salvarsan 606 was too painful to inject. Some doctors were worried about injecting the patients with arsenic, despite all Ehrlich's tests. Some doctors said that people would have sex with lots of different people now they knew that syphilis could be cured.

MALARIA

The Romans knew about malaria. They did not know what caused it, but they did know it was linked to swamps. The next stage in the long process of finding out the cause was when Charles Laveran discovered (in 1880) that tiny parasites were involved in passing on the disease.

It was known that parasites in mosquitoes passed on other diseases and that mosquitoes were to be found in swamps. In 1892 Dr Ronald Ross suggested that malaria was passed on by mosquitoes breeding in stagnant water. He did some research and proved this was the case. Once this was known, malaria was attacked by draining the places where malaria-carrying mosquitoes bred.

Sulphonamide drugs

Gerhard Domagk, another German scientist, admired Ehrlich's work. He wanted to find more magic bullets that would kill germs but not the sick person.

Germanin and prontosil

Domagk discovered germanin, a drug which worked against sleeping sickness. Then, in 1932, he discovered **prontosil**. This was made from a red dye and it killed the germ that caused blood poisoning. It worked on mice but he did not know if it would work on humans.

Then, in 1935, his daughter was injured by an infected needle. The wound turned bad and she was very ill with blood poisoning. Domagk gave her prontosil and she recovered.

What was in the prontosil?

Other scientists discovered that the important part of prontosil was sulphonamide made from coal tar.

Soon they made other medicines from sulphonamides. These medicines helped against diseases like scarlet fever, tonsillitis and pneumonia

Disadvantages of sulphonamides

Sulphonamides could damage a person's kidneys and liver. Also, they did not work against very strong germs. An even better magic bullet was needed.

The beginning of penicillin

Penicillin was the first **antibiotic**. It was the first drug made from living things like fungi. It stopped bacteria (germs) growing. Three people worked to discover it: **Alexander Fleming**, **Howard Florey** and **Ernst Chain**.

Stage 1 1928

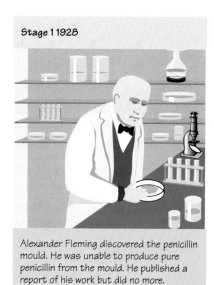

Alexander Fleming discovered the penicillin mould. He was unable to produce pure penicillin from the mould. He published a report of his work but did no more.

Stage 2 1938–41

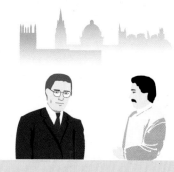

A team of researchers at Oxford University, led by Howard Florey and Ernst Chain, developed a method of making pure penicillin. They could not make large amounts however.

Stage 3 1941–44

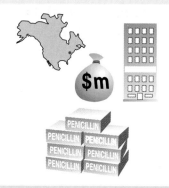

In 1941 the USA entered the Second World War. The US government funded research into methods of making large quantities of penicillin. By 1944 enough penicillin was available for Allied soldiers.

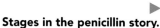

Stages in the penicillin story.

Alexander Fleming

Fleming was born in Scotland in 1881. In 1906 he went to study medicine at St. Mary's Hospital, London. He worked under **Sir Almroth Wright**, a very famous doctor.

When the First World War started, in 1914, Fleming worked in army hospitals in France. He was horrified to see that many soldiers with deep wounds died, because their wounds went bad. Nothing could save them.

After the First World War

By 1928, Fleming was studying **staphylococci** (germs which make wounds go bad). He grew the germs in little dishes.

One day he was cleaning out a dish when he noticed that some mould was growing in it. This often happened. But this time Fleming noticed that all around the mould, the germs had stopped growing!

Was the mould killing the germs?

Penicillin

Fleming grew more of the mould (*penicilium notatum*). He made a juice from the mould and called it penicillin , after the mould itself. This penicillin juice killed many deadly germs if he injected it into sick animals. The animals got better.

But no one was interested enough to give Fleming any money to make a pure drug for human beings.

In 1929 Fleming wrote an article about penicillin. He then stopped working on it. Nothing more happened for six years.

Source O

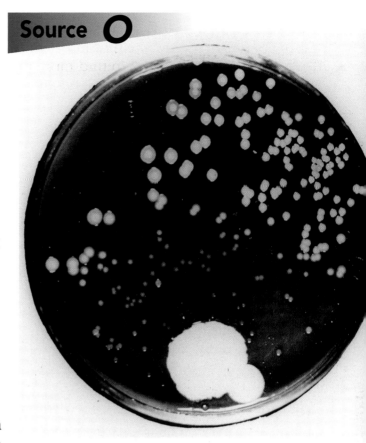

▲ The dish with the 'abnormal' culture. The mould is on the left. On the right, germs are growing, but near the mould there is a clear area.

Howard Florey and Ernst Chain

In 1935 Howard Florey headed a team of brilliant scientists at Oxford.

One of these scientists was Ernst Chain, a Jewish refugee from Nazi Germany. Chain read the old article written by Fleming all about penicillin.

Florey and Chain decided to try to make penicillin themselves. They managed to do this and tested it on sick mice. The mice got better. Florey said it was a miracle.

Problems of making pure penicillin

Florey and Chain grew the mould in milk bottles and bed pans. They had no money to make penicillin on a big scale.

But by 1940 they had made enough to treat a policeman who was dying from blood-poisoning. He got much better. Then the penicillin ran out and he died. But they had proved it worked.

The Second World War

Britain was fighting Germany. All the big chemical factories were making bombs and did not have time to try and make penicillin. So Florey went to the USA. Still no one would give him the money to make large amounts of penicillin.

Then, in 1941, the USA joined the war against Germany. The US government gave money to chemical firms so they could buy the equipment to make penicillin on a huge scale.

Penicillin saved many wounded soldiers lives in the Second World War.

Factors involved in penicillin

The penicillin story showed how a number of factors could work together to bring about an important discovery. These factors were:

- chance
- governments
- war
- research teams
- individual brilliance.

Fleming and the Nobel Prize

In 1942, Alexander Fleming's friend was dying. Fleming asked Florey if he could have some penicillin. Florey sent some and the friend got better. The story appeared in *The Times* newspaper, followed by a letter from Sir Almroth Wright (see Source Q). Suddenly, everyone began to say that Fleming *alone* had discovered penicillin. Florey and Chain and Fleming were given the **Nobel Prize** together in 1945. But it is Fleming who has become famous for discovering penicillin.

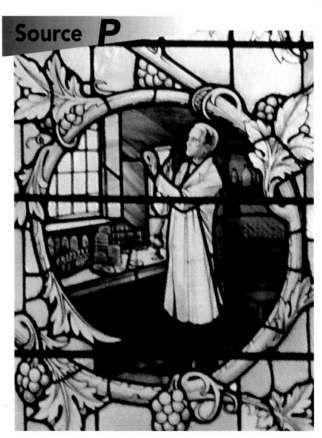

Source P

▲ A stained glass window, showing Alexander Fleming at work in his laboratory. It is in a church close to the hospital where Fleming worked for 49 years.

Professor Alexander Fleming of this laboratory is the discoverer of penicillin and also the author of the original suggestion that it might ...have important uses in medicine.

▲ From a letter written to *The Times* by Sir Almroth Wright, 30 August 1942.

Source *R*

There has been a lot in the newspapers and press about penicillin. It is presented as worked out by Fleming. Some scientists have now said to us, 'But I thought you had done something on penicillin too'.

▲ Extract from a letter written by Howard Florey to Sir Henry Dale in December 1942. Dale was the President of the Royal Society, a body concerned with the advancement of science and medicine.

NEW DISEASES

Since the 1940s a number of lethal diseases, thought to be new, have developed. The best known of these is AIDS. Others include Lassa fever, Creutzfeld-Jacob disease, Dengue and Ebola virus.

Research has shown that these are not new diseases at all. They are changed forms of old diseases. Viruses can become used to antibiotics. The antibiotics no longer work. When this happens, new antibiotics have to be developed. Some viruses can change before an antibiotic has been developed to fight them. Genetic engineering and biochemistry now play an important part in finding and fighting these viruses.

Has infectious disease been conquered?

Penicillin and other antibiotics have been very successful. Today, in Britain and other developed countries, few people die of infectious diseases. However, infectious diseases have not died out altogether.

- Tuberculosis killed 18 million people in 1990. (Most deaths were in the developing world.)
- Scientists are now searching for a vaccine for AIDS.
- Some germs have become immune to antibiotics such as penicillin.

Safety

Drug companies make a lot of money. They can be tempted to put drugs out that have not been fully tested. In 1964 the British Government set up the Committee on Safety of Drugs to check on testing.

SUMMARY

- ▶ **1891** Behring found a cure for diphtheria.
- ▶ **1909** Ehrlich and Hata discovered Salvarsan 606 which kills the syphilis germ.
- ▶ **1932** Domagk discovered prontosil, the first sulphonamide drug.
- ▶ **1928** Fleming discovered penicillin – the first antibiotic drug.
- ▶ **1938** Florey and Chain began to research penicillin.
- ▶ **1942** The chemical industry in the USA started to make penicillin on a big scale.

It is easy to forget the human guinea-pigs used to test new drugs, anaesthetics and surgical procedures. Some of them could afford to take the risk of testing a new drug. Joseph Meister (see page 86), just nine years old, had been bitten by a rabid dog while walking to school. He was rescued by a bricklayer who beat the dog off with an iron bar. But the boy had been bitten and was covered in blood and saliva. He would have died of rabies without Pasteur's vaccine. Sometimes a treatment (or drug) must be tried on a healthy person to prove that it works. Jenner had to test his vaccine by giving it to a healthy person, who he then deliberately infected with smallpox. It was a dangerous experiment. Maybe this is why Jenner chose James Phipps, the child of a poor family who lived nearby. Some experiments on human guinea-pigs succeeded. James Phipps and Joseph Meister both lived. Others failed. Some of the problems, dangers and frustrations of early research appear in the story of Albert Alexander, the policeman, told in the box on the right. New drugs and procedures are being tested all the time. They need human volunteers who all help the development of medicine.

Source 1

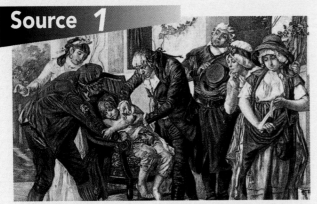

▲ An artist's interpretation of Jenner vaccinating James Phipps.

October 12, 1940 Policeman, aged 43 admitted. Suppuration of the face, scalp and both eye sockets, starting from a sore at the corner of the mouth a month earlier. Primary infection *staphylococcus aureus*. Secondary infection *streptococcus pyrogenes*.

December 12–19 Sulphapyridine, 19gr given; no improvement; drug rash.

January 19 Incision of multiple abscesses on face and scalp...

February 9 Blood transfusion, about 1 litre. Fever intermittent 98–101°F, very ill, emaciated; tongue heavily furred; right eye bulging, cut, pus has *staphylococcus*.

February 12 All incisions suppurating; scalp, face, eyes and right arm. Lungs involved. Penicillin 200mg given intravenously; then 100mg three-hourly, intravenous except for two intramusclar doses. Slight rigor after first dose, otherwise no reactions. Striking improvement after total of 800mg of penicillin in 24 hours. Cessation of scalp discharge, diminution of right eye suppuration. Arm discharge seemed less.

February 16 Much improvement; right eye almost normal. Some discharge still from the left eye and arm. Shortage of penicillin interrupted treatment from noon till 6pm; then drip infusion of 200mg.

February 17 Penicillin supply exhausted. Total administered 4.4g in 5 days. Patient much improved; no fever, appetite better, resolution of infections in face, scalp and right eye; still coughing; sputum contained *streptococcus pyrogenes*. Left eye still suppurating. Urine normal. Condition stationary for ten days, then deteriorated, especially lungs.

March 15 Patient died.

▲ From *The Lancet*, August 16, 1941.

CHAPTER 12

THE REVOLUTION IN SURGERY

12.1 Anaesthetics conquer pain

The problems of surgery
Surgeons had always faced three main problems:
pain, **infection** and **bleeding**.

The problem of pain
For hundreds of years there were no good pain-killers.
Surgeons cut off arms and legs or took out stones and
the patient screamed with pain. Often they died from
the shock of the pain.

Chemist discovers laughing gas
Humphrey Davy was a chemist. In 1799 he discovered
people did not feel pain if they breathed in **nitrous
oxide** (laughing gas). He wrote about his discovery
but surgeons ignored it.

FIGHTING PAIN

Anaesthetics are pain-
killing drugs. There are
two sorts:

General anaesthetics –
These make the patient
completely unconscious.

Local anaesthetics –
These stop pain in one
place, such as in a tooth.

Source A

Source B

A patient getting ready
for an operation was like
a prisoner condemmed
to death.

▲ Said in 1848, by someone
who had surgery before
effective anaesthetics.

◀ A cartoon of an operation
in 1793.

The search for a good anaesthetic

In 1842 Crawford Long used **ether** as a general anaesthetic. It worked but he did not tell anyone about it.

Nitrous oxide

Horace Wells was an American dentist. In 1845 he went to a fair and saw people breathing in nitrous oxide for fun. They laughed a lot. They also felt no pain at all. The next day Wells had a tooth out. He breathed nitrous oxide first. He felt no pain at all. But Wells did not know that some people are not affected by nitrous oxide. When he tried to show a group of students how to take a tooth out without pain, the patient shouted with pain.

Problems with nitrous oxide

Wells used nitrous oxide in several more operations where it worked. Then a patient died from being given too much. Wells killed himself. William Morton, Wells' partner, looked for a safer anaesthetic.

A safer anaesthetic – ether

Morton found that ether worked well. In 1846 he and John Warren cut a tumour off Gilbert Abbott's neck. They gave him ether first. He did not feel a thing.

Spreading the news

This time news spread fast. A doctor who had seen the operation on Abbot wrote an article about it the next week. He also wrote a letter to a friend in Britain. Steamships now crossed the Atlantic. They were faster than sailing ships. By 19 December 1846 the friend, Dr Boot, had the letter and had taken a tooth out using ether. On 21 December Robert Liston amputated a man's leg using ether.

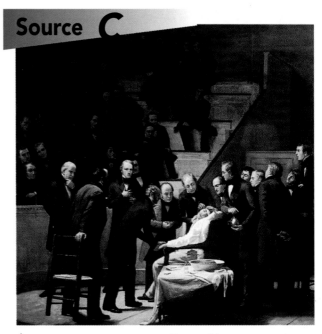

▲ Warren's operation on Gilbert Abbott, painted in 1882.

This Yankee dodge, gentlemen, beats mesmerism hollow!

▲ Said by Robert Liston to the people who had watched him operate in 1846.

QUESTIONS

1 Draw out a chart like the one below. Fill in the chart to show when experiments were made with anaesthetics.

Date	Event	Person(s) involved

2 Source C was painted long after the operation. Is it a reliable source of evidence for a historian? Give reasons for your answer.

Problems with ether

Ether could catch fire. It had a strong smell and made patients cough a lot.

James Young Simpson and chloroform

Simpson wanted to find a better anaesthetic than ether. He particularly wanted to help women with pain in childbirth. In 1847 he discovered that **chloroform** was easier to breathe in. Not very much was needed and it knocked people out quickly (see Source E).

Some people were against anaesthetics

- Some people thought doctors did not know how much to give or what side effects there might be. (Some patients did die of anaesthetics).

- Members of the Calvinist Church in Scotland said that the Bible said women were supposed to suffer pain in childbirth.

- Some people worried that surgeons could cut off whatever they liked while the patient was unconscious!

- Some army doctors thought using anaesthetics was 'soft'.

- There had been cases of ether exploding in the operating theatre.

Late one evening Dr. Simpson and his two friends sat down [to try out different anaesthetics].

Having sniffed several substances, Dr. Simpson decided to try one that he did not think was much use – a small bottle of chloroform. He found it under a pile of paper. [They breathed in the chloroform and passed out].

When he woke up Dr. Simpson thought, 'This is far stronger and better than ether.'

▲ From H. L. Gordon, *Sir James Young Simpson and Chloroform*, 1897.

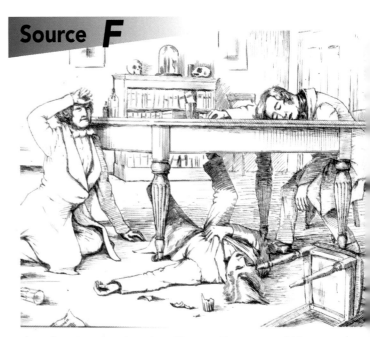

▲ A drawing showing the effect on Simpson and his friends of breathing in chloroform.

Queen Victoria and chloroform

Queen Victoria had chloroform for the birth of her eighth child in 1853. The Queen wrote that chloroform 'was soothing, quietening and delightful.' After this lots of people began to think it was a good idea. It was used a lot until 1900. Then it was discovered it could damage the liver. Surgeons went back to using ether.

Problems with anaesthetics

Anaesthetics were wonderful. For the first time in history patients could have operations without pain. But there were problems. Sometimes so much anaesthetic had to be used (to relax the muscles) that patients slept for days.

New anaesthetics

In 1884 cocaine was used as a local anaesthetic. Then, in 1905, novocaine was found to work better. In 1942 **curare**, a South American poison, was used to relax muscles and worked very well.

Anaesthetists today

Anaesthetists are specially skilled doctors. They give the anaesthetic. They monitor the heart beat, blood pressure, breathing and brain waves on high technology machines.

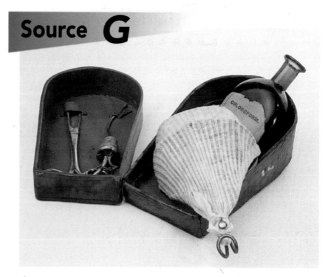

▲ An inhaler for breathing in chloroform from 1879.

ASPIRIN

Anaesthetics provided pain relief for surgery. Drugs were also being developed for the relief of more minor pain. Some of these drugs could trace their first use back to older herbal cures.

Aspirin contains salicylic acid, which is also present in willow leaves, which the Egyptians used to relieve pain.

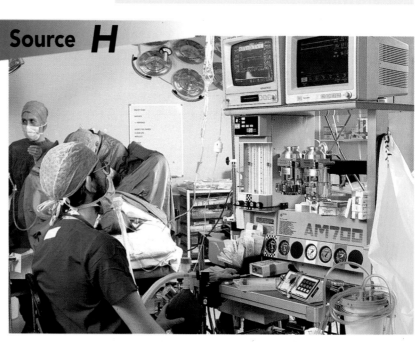

▶ Modern anaesthetists at work.

The problem of infection

From 1846 there were anaesthetics. So surgeons did a lot more operations. But still many patients died. The time from 1846–70 is sometimes called the **'black period'** of surgery. Surgeons wore old blood-stained clothes. They did not wash their hands or their knives. The trouble was surgeons did not know about germs.

Ignaz Semmelweiss and puerperal fever

Semmelweiss was a doctor in Vienna in the 1840s. He was worried that so many women died after childbirth from **puerperal fever**. They had the baby. They seemed to be weak but all right. Then they got a fever and died. In 1847 Semmelweiss said that he thought the fever was spread by the doctors themselves. Doctors dissected women who had died of puerperal fever. Then they went straight from the dissecting room to examine women who had just had a baby. They did not even wash their hands.

Semmelweiss ordered that all doctors working for him washed their hands in a solution of chloride of lime before they examined their patients. After this fewer women died but other doctors did not accept what Semmelweiss said.

Joseph Lister and antiseptics

Lister read about Pasteur's work on the germ theory. Lister realized that germs were killing his patients. He decided to kill the germs instead.

Carbolic acid

Lister used carbolic acid to kill germs. It is very strong. At first he soaked bandages in it. He found that the wounds did not go bad. But the patient was burned by the carbolic acid. Next he decided to use it as a spray. Everything in the operating theatre was sprayed with carbolic acid, including the surgeon's hands, the knives and the patient. Far fewer patients died.

JOSEPH LISTER
(1828–1912)

Lister was Professor of Surgery at Glasgow. Many doctors were against his ideas but it was soon obvious that his antiseptic carbolic acid worked.

The figures below come from his records of amputations. They show how useful antiseptics were.

Date	How many patients	How many died
1864–6 (no antiseptics)	35	16
1867–70 (antiseptics)	40	6

Source 1

Chance did not play a part in Lister's discovery. He had read of the germ theory and had applied it.

Millions of lives were saved by the new idea of antisepsis [the use of antiseptics to kill germs].

The frightful spectre [of death] which had haunted operating theatres had been shown to have a cause. Lister had shown how to defeat it.

▲ Adapted from *Microbes and Men* by Robert Reid, 1974.

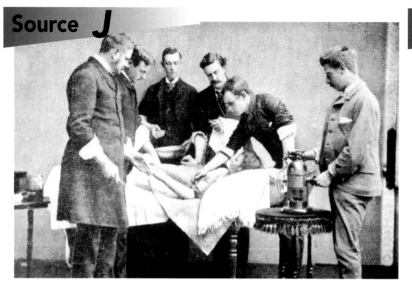

▲An operation in the 1880s. Lister's steam carbolic spray is being used.

Lots of people were against Lister and his ideas of antiseptics such as carbolic acid killing germs.

Fully twenty years were needed before British surgeons were won over to Lister's idea.

▲Adapted from Leo M. Zimmermann and Ilza Veith, *Great Ideas in the History of Surgery*, 1961.

Aseptic surgery (keeping clean)

Antiseptics such as carbolic acid burnt the skin. So surgeons in Germany decided to keep all germs out of operating theatres if they could. Everything was washed and sterilized. For instance, all the knives were sterilized by passing superheated steam over them. This was called **aseptic** surgery

Rubber gloves

William S. Halsted was a leading American surgeon. In 1889 his nurse (and future wife) complained that the antiseptic chemicals he used were ruining her hands. Halsted asked the Goodyear Rubber Company to make some rubber gloves she could wear. He quickly realized that these clean gloves also kept germs away from patients. Soon he made his team of doctors and nurses wear caps, masks and gowns for surgery.

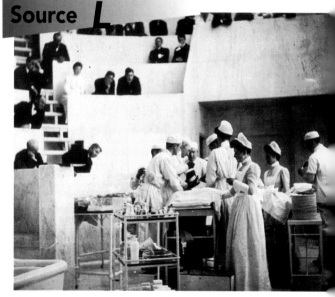

▲Halsted in the operating theatre. He operated and taught his students at the same time.

The problem of bleeding

A lot of blood can be lost during an operation. Doctors had tried for a long time to replace lost blood. They did not have much success. In 1667 in France a doctor had put blood from a lamb into a boy. The boy lived. But the next patient died. Much later, in 1818, doctors passed blood from one human to another but it usually did not work.

Blood groups

In 1900 Karl Landsteiner discovered that there were different **blood groups**. A patient who had lost a lot of blood had to have blood from someone who was of the same blood group. This discovery helped surgeons.

In the First World War (1914–1918) ways of storing blood were discovered. Then, in 1938, the National Blood Transfusion Service was set up in Britain. People gave blood. It was tested for blood group, stored and used when needed.

Plastic surgery

Surgeons in India and in Europe had patched skin for hundreds of years, but there was a chance it might go bad.

In the 20th century two world wars and new weapons meant that many people had bad injuries. In Britain Harold Gillies was the first plastic surgeon to work to help badly injured people look better.

In the Second World War, Gillies' assistant, Archibald McIndoe, set up a special hospital to treat patients (mostly airmen) who had been badly burned by petrol.

The use of the new drugs, sulphonamides and penicillin, helped him in his work by keeping infection down.

Source M

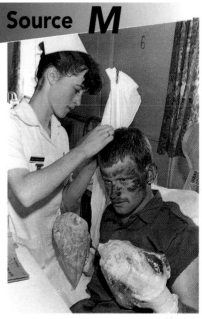

▲ **A serviceman with lots of burns being treated during the Falklands War, 1982.**

Source N

One hundred and fifty years ago, patients would only lie on the operating table if they were desperate with pain from their leg rotting or from bladder stones.

Now with anaesthesia, antiseptics, blood transfusion and antibiotics, everything is available for the surgeon's healing knife.

▲ **A comment by Professor Harold Ellis in the BBC television programme, *The Courage to Fail*, in 1987.**

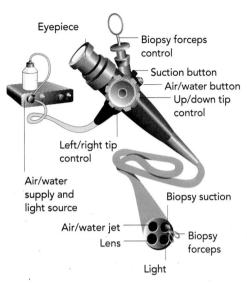

Endoscopes using fibre optics can examine almost every hollow tube in the body.

Labels for diagram: Eyepiece, Biopsy forceps control, Suction button, Air/water button, Up/down tip control, Left/right tip control, Air/water supply and light source, Biopsy suction, Air/water jet, Lens, Biopsy forceps, Light

Discoveries that have helped surgery since 1895

X-rays: In 1895 Wilhelm Röntgen discovered X-rays. Surgeons could see pictures of the inside of a person's body without cutting them open.

Radium: In 1898 Marie and Pierre Curie discovered radium. This later helped to treat cancer.

Electrocardiograph: In 1903 Willem Einthoven developed electrocardiographs. These monitored the heartbeat.

Artificial kidney machine: In 1943 a Dutch surgeon, Willem Kolff made the first artificial kidney machine.

Heart-lung machine: In 1953 a heart-lung machine was used in an operation. The patient's heart was stopped for some time. The machine took over. This gave the surgeons more time to operate.

Microsurgery: In the 1960s new microscopes, fine needles and threads meant surgeons could sew up tiny nerves and blood vessels (as in sewing on a finger).

Fibre optics: Today fibre optics mean that surgeons can see inside the body by putting fine tubes through the mouth or rectum, or through a keyhole sized cut.

Keyhole surgery: Today tiny cuts can be made to take out things like the gall bladder. Patients get better more quickly.

New plastics and steel: Today new joints for the body can be made of plastic or steel.

Source O

During the mid-1960s, I remember wards having forty beds.

They had a family feeling because after an operation patients spent seven to ten days there and got to know each other.

The surgeon and anaesthetist would often parade around the ward to see that all was well. No one changed out of their bloodstained surgical gowns.

During visiting time we packed and sterilized the instruments for the operations on the next day.

Denise Simpson remembers her first years as a nurse.

A surgeon using an endoscope (fibre optics) to look inside the patient.

Source P

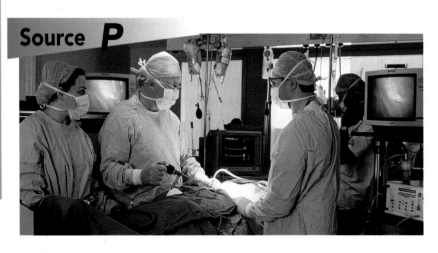

Heart surgery

Before the Second World War no one operated on hearts. As soon as the chest was cut open, the lungs collapsed. If the heart was touched it stopped.

The Second World War

An American surgeon, Dwight Harken, came across many soldiers with bullets or bits of shrapnel in their hearts. He tried to save them. He cut into the beating heart and hooked out the bullet with his fingers.

The main problem with cutting into the heart was that the blood supply had to be stopped. A surgeon only had four minutes to operate. The brain was damaged if the blood supply was stopped for more than four minutes.

The 1960s

Several surgeons started to work on heart surgery. They were helped by the heart-lung machine (see page 102). Many surgeons wanted to find a way to replace a sick heart with a healthy one (perhaps from someone killed in a road accident).

Christiaan Barnard

Christiaan Barnard was the first surgeon to **transplant** a heart from one body to another (see box).

Source Q

Of the first group all the patients died. In the second group half died. In the third group two out of the fourteen died. In the fourth group all the patients lived. The first three groups were animals, the fourth group were injured soldiers.

▲ **Dwight Harken's operations on injured hearts.**

Source R

Administrators said we were spending too much. They had the stupidity to say that, if we kept patients out, we could work within budget. I said, 'No problem. We've got a shot gun. I'll load it. You fire it, because that's what you're planning. Now, out.'

▲ **A British heart surgeon, describing the problems of getting money for operations in the 1960s.**

Source S

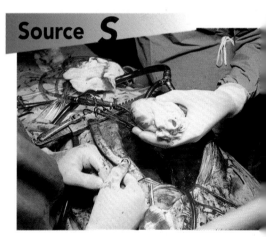

▲ **New discoveries meant heart-lung machines let surgeons work on the heart.**

CHRISTIAAN BARNARD

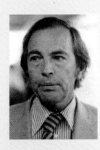

Christiaan Barnard trained in heart surgery in the USA. Working in South Africa he transplanted the heart of a woman who had died in a road accident into 59 year-old Louis Washkansky. Washkansky lived for eighteen days but then died of pneumonia. He was on special drugs to stop his body rejecting the new heart. The drugs stopped his body fighting the pneumonia.

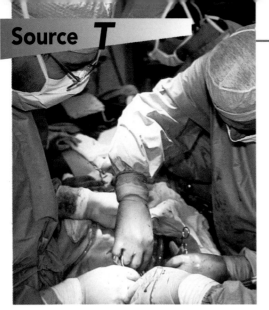

▲ **An open heart operation. The heart-lung machine is doing the work of the heart.**

Problems with heart transplants

There was one great problem with heart transplants. The patients bodies' wanted to kill the alien heart. To stop this happening the patients were given very strong drugs. These drugs killed the antibodies that attacked the new alien heart. So far, so good. However, the drugs also killed all the antibodies that kept out diseases like colds, 'flu and pneumonia. So patients woke up from their operations with new hearts but soon died of some other disease.

Artificial hearts

Transplants were given up and some surgeons tried artificial hearts but without much success.

A new breakthrough – cyclosporin

By chance someone discovered a new antibiotic in 1974. It stopped antibodies attacking a new heart but it did not kill off all the antibodies. Transplants were possible again. By 1987, ninety per cent of patients with transplants lived for two years or more. Transplants are now done regularly.

SUMMARY

► Anaesthetics and antiseptics made surgery safer after 1870.

► Aseptic surgery (no germs in the operating theatre) took over from antiseptic surgery.

► The discovery of different blood groups allowed blood transfusions.

► Surgeons specialized – in plastic surgery, heart surgery and so on.

► Science helped with new discoveries in plastics, X-rays and machines.

► Wars in the 20th century speeded up developments in surgery.

HELEN TAUSSIG

Dr Helen Taussig (1898–1986) went to Johns Hopkins Medical School in 1921. By 1938 she was a world expert in inherited heart disease.

Taussig studied the problem of 'blue babies'. These babies were born with defective hearts. Their skin was blue through lack of oxygen. She felt that if the narrow valves of the heart could be bypassed the babies would recover. She worked out an operation that would do this. The babies were kept alive. Many of them survived until an operation was developed to repair their hearts.

In 1962 Taussig led an investigation into Thalidomide, a drug which caused deformity. It was then banned.

Nursing before 1850

Many women nursed their families when they were sick. But there was no training for nurses. Paid nurses worked by common sense and what they had learnt from others. Some had a bad reputation for drinking and being dirty.

In the 1850s a German doctor ran a small hospital at Kaiserwerth. He insisted on a good standard of nursing. Elizabeth Fry set up a school for nurses in England after she had visited the hospital at Kaiserwerth.

Florence Nightingale (1820–1910)

Florence Nightingale wanted to be a nurse. It took her seven years to persuade her parents to let her do this. She visited Kaiserwerth and then studied nursing in Paris. In 1853 she ran the Institution for the Care of Sick Gentlewomen in London.

The Crimean War (1854–56)

Britain went to war against Russia in a place called the Crimea. There were many battles. Soldiers were dying in dirty, crowded hospitals at places such as **Scutari**.

Florence Nightingale at Scutari

The British Secretary for War was a friend of the Nightingale family. He asked if Florence would go out to Scutari. He wanted her to organize the hospital there. Florence sailed for Scutari with 38 nurses she had chosen.

The army doctors did not like all these female nurses arriving. But Nightingale was a good organizer. She obtained better water supplies and better food. She made sure that the wards were kept clean and that there were plenty of bandages. The death rate dropped from 42 per cent to 2 per cent.

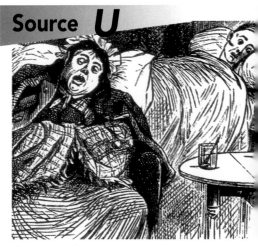

Source U

▲ This illustration shows how nurses were pictured in the first half of the 19th century – old, ugly and probably drunk.

Source V

She was a woman of iron will. She had friends in the government. She was determined to improve nursing education and care. She succeeded.

The organization of medical and nursing services everywhere, owe something to her spirit.

▲ Adapted from Philip Rhodes, *An Outline History of Medicine*, 1985.

Source W

Mary Seacole was a wonderful woman ...All the men asked her advice and used her herbal medicines rather than report to the doctors. She always helped the wounded after a battle and this made her loved by the whole army.

▲ From the memories of a British soldier who fought in the Crimean War.

Mary Seacole (1805–81)

Mary Seacole was born in Jamaica. Her mother ran a home for sick soldiers. Mary helped her mother look after the patients.

The Crimean War

Seacole went to Britain and asked to go out to the Crimea as a nurse. She was rejected. She did not give up. She sailed for the Crimea (paying for her own ticket).

She set up a medical store, and looked after soldiers on the battlefield too. Seacole met Florence Nightingale, who would not take her on as a nurse.

After the Crimean War

Mary Seacole went back to Britain but no one thanked her for the work she had done. She went bankrupt.

Then the newspapers took up her story. Some money was raised to help her and she wrote her life story to raise money too.

Source X

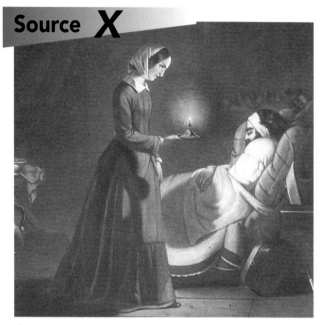

▲ Florence Nightingale became known as 'the lady with the lamp'. This picture was painted by Tomkins in 1855.

Source Y

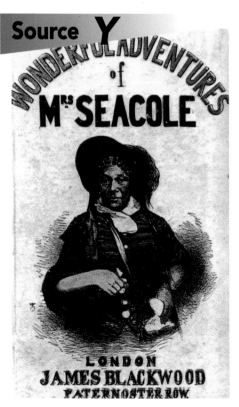

▲ A picture of Mary Seacole from her autobiography, *The Wonderful Adventures of Mrs Seacole*, 1857.

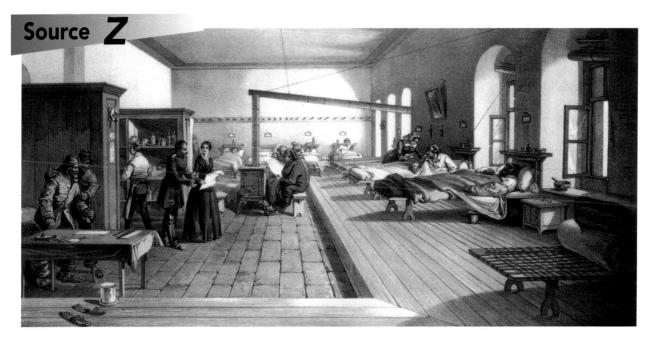

▲ The hospital at Scutari, after it had been cleaned and reorganized by Nightingale nurses.

The rise of nursing

On her return to England Florence Nightingale became very famous. She wrote a book called *Notes on Nursing*, describing her method of nursing. Nightingale wanted to train more women to be nurses. A lot of money was raised for her.

The money was used to set up the Nightingale School of Nursing at St. Thomas's Hospital in London.

Good Nursing

Florence Nightingale said that hospitals must be kept clean and nurses must work very hard and be well trained. Each nurse trained for three years.

Very soon other training schools were set up. By 1900 there were 64,000 trained nurses in Britain.

In 1919 the government passed an Act which laid down qualifications needed to become a nurse.

NURSING THE POOR

William Rathbone, a rich Liverpool trader, was an important person in the development of nursing for the poor in the late 19th century. He and Florence Nightingale set up a school in the Liverpool Royal Infirmary to train district nurses who would visit the sick in their homes. By 1887 nearly all large British cities were using district nurses.

Rathbone also started the reform of nursing conditions in workhouses. He influenced changes in the Poor Law that provided workhouses with better medical services.

ELIZABETH GARRETT ANDERSON
(1836–1917)

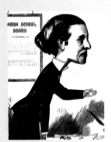

She trained as a nurse then wanted to be a doctor. No medical school would let her train as a doctor. In the end she trained privately. In 1865 she was accepted as a doctor by the Society of Apothecaries and soon had a large practice in London.

A hundred and fifty years ago men did not allow women to go to university. In 1849 a women did become a doctor in the USA. But in Britain male doctors were very much against women. They said women were 'too emotional' to be doctors.

Things begin to change

In the 1860s some people began to say that women should have the same rights as men.

The first women doctors

Elizabeth Garrett Anderson and Sophia Jex-Blake were the first women to become doctors.

The Sex Discrimination Act 1975

Through the 20th century more and more women trained as doctors. Then, in 1975, a law was passed in Parliament. It said that all jobs were open to women and men on the same terms.

SOPHIA JEX-BLAKE
(1840–1912)

In 1869 Sophia and four other women started to train as doctors at Edinburgh University. Then there was a law case and they were told it was against the law for them to train. Sophia got her medical degree in Switzerland. Then she set up the London School of Medicine for Women in 1874. She was the first woman to practice as a doctor in Scotland.

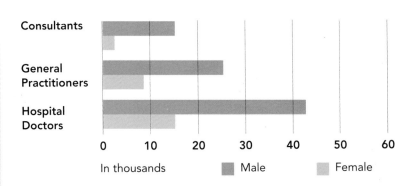

▲ Women doctors employed in the National Health Service in 1989.

PAULINE CUTTING

Pauline Cutting was a doctor in Beirut in 1987, when Palestinian refugees were under siege. There was no electricity, little food, no drugs, and bombing all the time. She stayed, worked on and saved many lives.

12.6 Case study: opposition to surgical progress

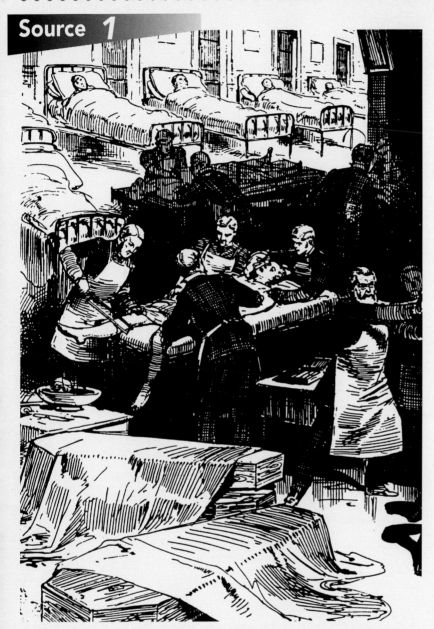

▲ This cartoon was called 'Operation Madness'. It was published in the 1870s. Anaesthetics had come into general use about this time. As there are coffins piled near to the operating table, the artist is quite clearly suggesting that the increase in the number of operations because of the use of anaesthetics will lead to certain death.

Anaesthetics allowed surgeons to attempt operations that they would never previously have dared to do. Unluckily, post-operative infection killed many of the patients. In Paris sixty per cent of those operated on died. In Edinburgh it was forty three per cent. In America, one proud surgeon announced that only a quarter of his patients died after their operations.

There was, not surprisingly, loud opposition to surgery. The cartoon on the left is just one example of this opposition. Even Lister's discovery of antiseptic surgery did not silence the opposition. He found it hard to persuade people to try his methods. As late as 1882, Lawson Tait, a well known surgeon, recommended that 'a system of washing is much better [than carbolic acid spray]. I fill the abdomen with warm water and wash all the organs. The water is plain unfiltered tap water and has not been boiled.' But by 1900 most surgeons were convinced by the results of antisepsis. One French surgeon told Lister 'you have driven back death itself.'

CHAPTER 13

DEVELOPMENTS IN PUBLIC HEALTH

13.1 Public health up to 1850

Towns get bigger

From the late 18th century, more and more people were born and survived childhood diseases. Many of them went to work in the new factories. This meant that more houses were built around factories. So towns grew bigger and bigger.

The houses were crowded together. There were no pipes to take the sewage away. Many of the towns were filthy.

Smoke from factories

The new factories made woollen cloth, cotton, iron machinery and so on. They used coal to make power to run the machines. Smoke and fumes belched out of the chimneys.

The government did nothing to improve the living conditions in the towns. They were very unhealthy places indeed.

THE GROWTH OF TOWNS 1801–1901 (in thousands)			
City	1801	1851	1901
Birmingham	71	233	523
Bradford	13	104	280
Leeds	53	172	429
Liverpool	82	376	704
Manchester	70	303	645
Newcastle	33	88	247
Nottingham	29	57	240
Sheffield	46	135	407

Source A

Alfred and Beckwith Row are surrounded by an open drain. The houses have common, open privies [toilets] which are in the most offensive condition.

In one house I found six persons living in a very small room, two in bed, ill with fever.

In the same room a woman was working as a silk weaver.

▲ Bethnal Green, London, described by Dr Thomas Southwood-Smith in 1838.

▼ Manchester in about 1854.

Source B

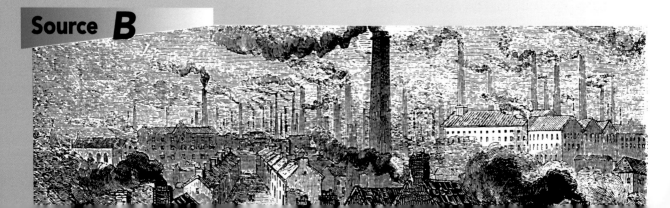

Dirt and disease

Where there was dirt there was disease. **Typhoid** was spread by dirty water. Typhus was spread by the bites from body lice.

Dirty living and poor food meant that people were less strong. They easily caught other diseases like smallpox and tuberculosis.

Cholera

In 1831 a new disease reached Britain. It was called **cholera.** So many people died that the government gave orders about burying people quickly.

By the end of 1832, cholera had spread over most of the country. About 21,000 people had died. Then the disease seemed to die out. But it came back again in 1848, 1854 and 1866.

The cause of cholera

No one knew what caused cholera at the time. Some people thought it was spread by poisonous gases in the air. Barrels of tar were burnt in the streets to try and 'purify' the air.

Now we know it was caused by a germ. This germ attacks the intestines. The sick person gets diarrhoea, vomiting, fever and soon dies.

Cholera is spread through water that is infected by the sewage from people with cholera.

▶ A memorial to 420 cholera victims in Dumfries, Scotland, 1832.

Source C

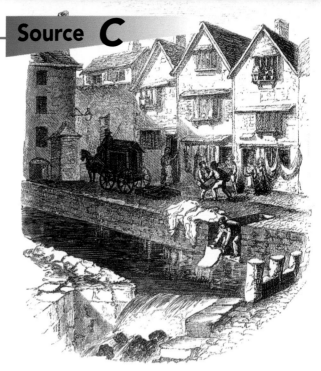

▲ Washing the dirty bedclothes of someone who had cholera, 1832. The stream was where most people got their drinking water.

Source D

Families huddled together in dirty rooms. There are slaughter houses in Butcher Row with rotting heaps of offal. Lots of pigs are kept. Chickens are kept in cellars. There are dung heaps everywhere.

▲ From *The History of the Cholera in Exeter in 1832,* written by Dr Thomas Shapter, in 1841.

Source E

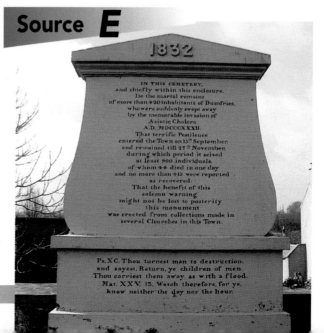

Edwin Chadwick

Everyone was shocked by the cholera epidemic of 1832. Something had to be done.

The government asked Edwin Chadwick to write a report about how poor people lived. The report came out in 1842. It said that many people in Britain were living in filthy and overcrowded houses.

Many people, including the rich, were horrified by Chadwick's report.

Source F

In one part of Market Street there is a dunghill. Yet it is too large to be called a dunghill. It is filth from all over the town. The person who deals in the dung sells it by the cartload.

This place is horrible, with swarms of flies which give a strong taste of the dunghill to any food left uncovered.

▲ This was written by Dr Laurie for Chadwick's report. It is about Greenock in Scotland.

Source G

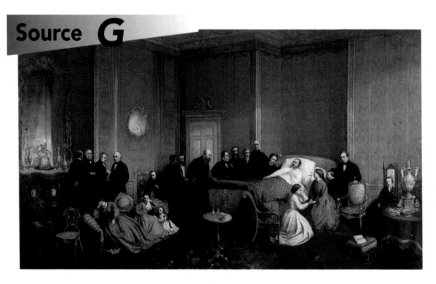

EDWIN CHADWICK
1800–90

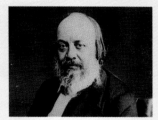

Chadwick was a lawyer.

He began to work for the government in 1832. He wrote a long report on the way poor people lived in Britain. It was called *A Report on the Sanitary Condition of the Labouring Population*. The report showed what terrible conditions many people lived in.

Chadwick said that if the towns were cleaner, there would be less disease. Then people would not need to take time off work.

Chadwick said that Parliament should pass laws to clean up towns. There should be pipes to take sewage away from houses. There should be pipes to bring clean water to houses.

Chadwick's work inspired the sanitary reform movement.

◄ The death of Prince Albert, Queen Victoria's husband. He died of typhoid fever in 1861. Windsor Castle had piped water. But the water was piped from the River Thames, which was filthy.

The Clean Party

After Chadwick's report a lot of people said that towns must be cleaned up.

They said that Parliament must pass a law saying that towns must have clean water for everyone. All the sewage must be taken away.

The Dirty Party

In 1847 a Public Health Bill was read in Parliament. Some people were against it.

They said that it was not the government's job to clean up towns. People should do it for themselves. If the government cleaned up the towns it would cost a lot of money. It would also mean that the government was poking its nose into everyone's business.

This way of thinking was called *laissez-faire* ('leave things alone' in French).

Cholera again 1848

Cholera struck again in 1848. Thousands died in the dirty towns. Suddenly, everyone wanted a clean up. The Public Health Act was made law in 1848.

The First Public Health Act 1848

Central Board of Health in London to sit for five years.

Local Boards of Health could be set up in towns if 10% of the rate payers agreed. These boards had the power to improve water supply and sewage disposals. They took over from private companies and individuals.

The Act was not compulsory. It was not fully applied across the whole country.

▲ **The terms of the first Public Health Act, 1848.**

Source H

Chadwick said that diseases such as cholera were caused by the rotting filth in towns. The towns should be cleaned up. The most important things were:

- good drains
- taking away rubbish
- clean water supplies.

'This expense would be a financial gain by lessening the cost of sickness and death.'

▲ **The main ideas from Chadwick's Report of 1842.**

Source I

Those against the Leeds Sewerage Scheme wanted to save the pockets of the ratepayers. Their idea was that the sewers were to discharge into the river nearby, thus carrying on the pollution.

▲ **Adapted from *Report on the Condition of the Town of Leeds*, 1844.**

TYPHOID

Typhoid fever was a deadly disease. It was often just called 'fever' or 'ague'. During the Crimean War (1854–6) it killed off ten times as many British soldiers as the enemy did.

By 1898 Almroth Wright had found a vaccine for the disease. It could be stopped but not cured. In 1900, in the Boer War, typhoid still killed more British soldiers than the enemy did.

The 1848 Public Health Act

This law said that towns could set up **Boards of Health** to clean up towns. But they did not have to. So only 182 towns did anything about cleaning up their water supplies and sewage.

Laissez-faire again

Some people still did not want the government to poke its nose into people's houses and streets, however dirty. Some rich people did not want to pay taxes to clean up poor parts of the towns.

Showing how cholera spread

Dr John Snow worked in London near Broad Street. He asked lots of people where they obtained their water. He noticed that all the people who caught cholera took their water from a pump in Broad Street. He took the handle off the pump. No one caught cholera. He showed that cholera was spread by infected water.

Chadwick and doctors

Chadwick said that everyone could be healthy if they had a clean place to live. He did not think much of doctors or hospitals. Some doctors disagreed with him. **Sir John Simon**, who was made Medical Officer for Health in 1858, did. He said you need a clean place to live and you need good doctors as well.

The government takes action

By 1872 the government realized that it had to do more about cleaning up towns. An Act of 1872 divided Britain into different areas. Each area had a Medical Officer of Health. A second Public Health Act was passed in 1875. This said that local town councils must provide clean water. In the same year an Act was passed saying that decent houses should be built for the workers. Britain was on its way to becoming a cleaner place.

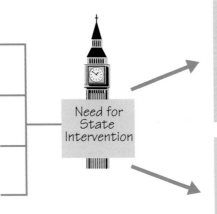

- Further cholera outbreaks in 1854 and 1866 frighten the authorities once more.
- In 1854 Dr John Snow showed that cholera was spread by contaminated water.
- In 1864 Louis Pasteur demonstrated the germ theory of disease. Need for cleanliness became clear.
- By the 1870s statistics showed that poor living conditions and disease were connected.

Need for State Intervention

1875 Second Public Health Act
- brought together all previous laws under one act.
- councils compelled to provide street lighting, clean water, drainage, and sewage disposal.
- councils had to employ medical inspectors.

1875 Artisans' Dwellings Act
- councils given power to buy up areas of slum housing, knock them down and build new houses.
- few councils took advantage.

▲ **Factors leading to state intervention into public health.**

Finding out about the poor

Charles Booth investigated how people lived in the East End of London.

He asked a lot of questions and wrote a book called *Life and Labour of the People in London*.

He said that one-third of the people lived below the poverty line. That is to say they did not have enough money to eat properly. They lived in bad houses. If they fell ill they could not afford to pay a doctor. People were poor because of sickness, old age, low wages or unemployment.

Seebohm Rowntree asked the same sort of questions in York. He found the same sort of answers as Booth had.

The Boer War 1899–1902

Then came the Boer War. Nearly half the men who wanted to join the army were unfit. They had grown up without enough food to eat. People were shocked.

The work of the Liberals 1906–14

The Liberal government was in power from 1906. They said something must be done to help poor people. One Liberal, **Winston Churchill**, said that the government had a duty to look after children, the sick and the elderly.

The box shows the laws that the Liberal government passed.

Source J

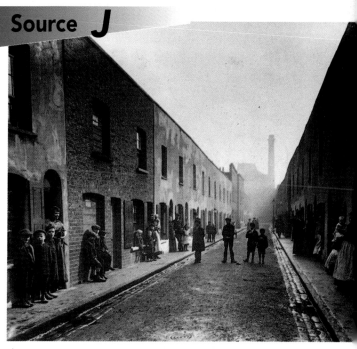

▲ Slum housing in the east end of London in 1912.

Date	Legislation
1906	**Provision of school meals** – local authorities given the power to provide free school meals.
1907	**School medical inspections.**
1909	**Old Age Pension Act** – people over 70 to receive 5s [25p] per week state pension as long as their income from other sources was not more than 12s [60p] per week.
1909	**Labour Exchanges** set up to help unemployed find work.
1911	**National Insurance Act** – two parts: Part I: Workers in manual trades earning less than £160 per year to pay 4d [2p] per week. The employer added 3d [1½p] and the government 2d [1p]. Workers entitled to 10s [50p] per week if they were off work sick, for up to 26 weeks. Free medical treatment available from a panel doctor. Part II: Workers, earning less than £160 per year in certain trades, together with the government and employers paid in 2½d [1p] per week. Workers could claim 7s [35p] unemployment pay for up to 15 weeks.

▲ Laws passed by the Liberal government 1906–14.

People against the new laws

Some people did not like the new laws. They said that people should be independent. They should not have old age pensions given to them. Rich people knew that the old age pensions would be paid for out of taxes paid by the better off. The rich did not want to pay more taxes.

In 1911 a National Insurance Act was passed (see box on page 115). This gave money to some workers if they could not work because they were sick or unemployed. Again some people said that workers should be more independent.

David Lloyd George

David Lloyd George was a leading member of the Liberal government. He pushed through many of the laws and said that this was only a start. There was a lot further to go to help poor people.

More laws 1919–39

After the First World War (1914–18) Lloyd George said he would make Britain 'a country fit for heroes to live in'.

In 1919 the Ministry of Health was set up. It was to deal with everything to do with health in Britain.

Also in 1919 a new law was passed to get more houses built for poorer people.

In 1920 another National Insurance Act was passed. The number of workers who were paid money because they were sick or unemployed was increased. Now only farm workers and servants were not covered.

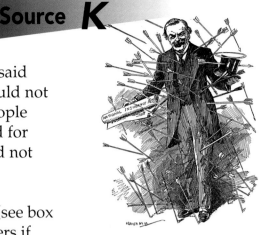

▲ Lots of people were against Lloyd George and his National Insurance Act. Do you think the cartoonist was for or against Lloyd George?

CRAPPER

Thomas Crapper was one of the many inventors and makers of toilets, baths and washbasins who set up after the 1848 Public Health Act.

The Act had said that every house should have a way of getting rid of sewage – a toilet and a drain to a sewer. First, of course, cities needed sewers. London's sewers were finished in 1865 – over 1,000 miles of them!

Crapper made toilets from his works in London. His *Improved Registered Ornamental Flush-down W.C.* cost £6.15s.0d (£6.75p).

It was Crapper who was asked to supply toilets for Sandringham, Norfolk, when it became a home for the royal family.

Bad times

Throughout the 1920s and 1930s the government was short of money. But, even so, a Pensions Act was passed in 1925. This said people should receive a pension when they were 65 years old.

Then there was a trade depression in the 1930s. Many people were unemployed. The government had to spend a lot of money on dole payments. There was not enough money left for anything else.

Many people still said that the government must do more about health. While the government (local authorities) did do some things about health, other things were done by volunteers. The whole set up was a muddle. For instance, the government provided 2,000 hospitals but there were also another 1,000 hospitals paid for by voluntary funds (see diagram below).

The Second World War broke out in 1939. It changed people's attitudes towards health care.

Source **L**

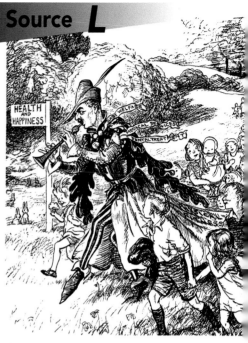

▲ This cartoon shows a member of the government wanting to lead the way to more laws about health.

An unco-ordinated system

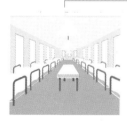

Hospitals
- About 3,000 in Britain, 1,000 were run by voluntary funds. Hospitals unevenly spread.
- Poor people were treated in workhouse infirmaries.

Doctors
- Wealthy received best treatment as they could afford the fees.
- Some workers, covered by National Insurance, had panel doctors. [dependants not covered]

Other services
Local authorities provided:
- school medical inspectors
- ante-natal clinics
- infant-welfare centres.

▲ Health care in 1939.

Source **M**

In 1939 most workers [but not their wives or children] were covered by social insurance schemes.

There were state schools and hospitals. There were ante-natal clinics and infant welfare clinics. Three million children got free milk in school.

▲ Adapted from Paul Addison, *A New Jerusalem*, 1994.

The Second World War

In the early months of the war, children were sent out of the cities to live in the country. Many people in the country were shocked at how poor these children were. Then the cities were bombed. Many people were injured. The government set up hospitals and free treatment. This worked very well.

The Beveridge Report 1942

William Beveridge wanted a **welfare state** where, the government helped people 'from the cradle to the grave.' In 1942 he published *The Beveridge Report*. In it he said he wanted everyone to be free from the five 'giants'. These were:

- Want (not enough money to live a healthy life)
- Disease
- Ignorance (everyone to have a chance to go to school)
- Squalor (filthy houses)
- Idleness (no work).

The Beveridge Report became a best seller. People wanted a better life for everyone after the war. Only people like Winston Churchill asked how it was to be paid for.

The Labour Government 1945–51

In July 1945 the Labour government came to power. They passed many laws to help poorer people. The most important was the setting up the **National Health Service** (NHS).

The National Health Service

The National Health Service started in 1948. It was the idea of **Aneurin Bevan**. It provided lots of things free.

- Hospitals
- Doctors and dentists
- Opticians
- Ambulances
- Vaccinations
- Health visitors and maternity clinics

Some doctors did not want to work for the government. So as well as being paid a fee (by the government) for each patient, they could treat private patients too.

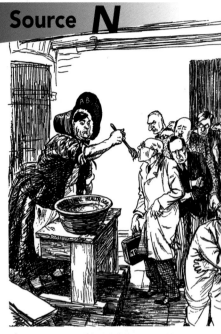

Source N

▲ **Aneurin Bevan dishes out NHS 'medicine' to the doctors. Many doctors did not want to work for the NHS at first.**

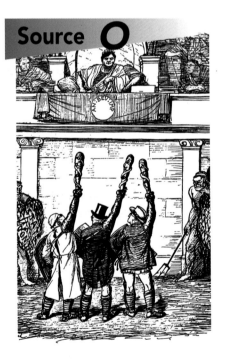

Source O

▲ **This cartoon from 1948 shows the government as a Roman Emperor and three doctors as gladiators. The Latin says 'We who are about to die, salute you'.**

The cost of the National Health Service

Most people thought the National Health Service was wonderful. But it did cost a lot of money. By 1950 it was costing the government (taxpayers) £350 million a year. This was twice as much as had been expected. The government brought in **prescription charges**.

The Introduction of Free Vaccinations in Britain	
1840	Smallpox
1948	Tuberculosis
1954	Diphtheria, whooping cough and tetanus ('triple vaccine')
1955	Polio
1964	Measles
1969	Rubella (German measles)

Vaccination

The government paid for the vaccination of all children (see box). Polio was a dreaded disease. It usually struck young people and could paralyse them for life. **Jonas Salk** found a vaccine in 1954. The government paid for this, too.

World Health Organization

This was set up in 1948. It was to help everyone in the world to be healthier. One of the things it did was to get more and more children vaccinated. Today eight out of ten children have been vaccinated against the worst diseases.

Alternative medicine

For the last 140 years one type of medicine has dominated. But many people have begun to worry that some of the powerful drugs can harm the body. This is particularly so if they are taken for a long time. Many drugs, such as painkillers, cover up the illness rather than cure it. More people are looking at other methods of healing. Illnesses like depression, arthritis and asthma can respond very well to treatments such as homeopathy (which uses 'natural' cures from plants and metals), acupuncture and faith healing (a spiritual cure).

Source P

She went and got tested for new glasses, then she went to the chiropodist, she had her feet done. Then she went back to the doctor's. He fixed her up with a hearing aid.

▲ From Paul Addison, *Now the War is Over*, 1985.

Source Q

The Times said that British people might get so used to having things served up on a plate that they would no longer help themselves.

▲ R. J. Cootes, *The Welfare State*, 1970.

Source R

The NHS started. My mother and dad had problems with their teeth and I think they were first at the dentist. And instead of having just a few teeth out they had the complete set. And free dentures. Thought it was wonderful.

▲ A woman describing her reaction to the NHS.

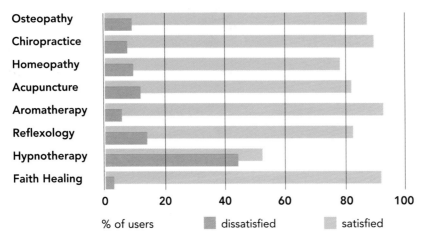

Osteopathy
Chiropractice
Homeopathy
Acupuncture
Aromatherapy
Reflexology
Hypnotherapy
Faith Healing

% of users ■ dissatisfied ■ satisfied

▲ A recent survey by the magazine, *Which*. People who had tried alternative treatments mainly saw them as successful.

Changes in the NHS

The cost of a free health service is enormous. More people are living longer. More illnesses can be treated today than could be treated 50 years ago.

In the 1980s the government encouraged people to take out private health insurance. But a lot of people said that then rich people would get better treatment than poorer people. Then the government said that hospitals must only have a certain amount of money. They had to stick to their **budget** and not overspend. This could mean that they might have to turn patients away.

ANEURIN BEVAN

Aneurin Bevan (1897–1960) was the Minister for Health who pushed for the setting up of the National Health Service (NHS).

Bevan was a firm believer in the welfare state. He thought that everyone should have free medical care. It was Bevan who persuaded senior medical staff in hospitals to agree to work within the NHS.

Bevan preferred to work by persuading people, not bullying them. Once he had persuaded the hospitals, he had to convince family doctors they should join the NHS.

By 1948 many doctors (even those who did not agree with his political ideas) saw that he was a person who was pepared to discuss things. Most of them followed the lead of the hospital doctors and joined the NHS system.

SUMMARY

▶ In the 19th century the government started to take more responsibility for public health.

▶ The Liberal government passed many laws to help poorer people. These laws included the Old Age Pensions Act in 1908.

▶ A few laws to help health were passed between 1919 and 1939. But mostly the government was worried about unemployment.

▶ *The Beveridge Report* (1942) said that everyone should be looked after 'from the cradle to the grave'.

▶ The National Health Service was started in 1948.

▶ The enormous cost of the National Health Service has made the government look again at how it is organized.

Pollution is not just a modern problem. Sewage and rubbish had always been dumped in rivers. On 21 August, 1841, a civil engineer wrote to a Leeds newspaper about water pollution in the River Aire:
The river is charged with the contents of about 200 lavatories and similar places, a great number of common drains, the drainings of dung hills, the Infirmary (dead leeches, poltices for patients etc.), slaughterhouses, chemicals, soap, gas, dung, dyehouses, factories, spent blue and black dye, pig manure, decomposed animal and vegetable substances. This amounts to about 30,000 gallons of filth a year.

As well as water, the air was also polluted. In 1852 Thomas Miller described London fog:
You imagine that all the smoke which had ascended for years from the thousands of London chimneys had fallen down at once after having rotted somewhere above the clouds.

The worst problems of sewage and polluted drinking water were largely solved by 1900. The problems of air pollution, dirty rivers and overcrowding were not. Indeed chemicals or radiation in the air, chemical or fertilizer spills into rivers and inadequate housing still constitute health hazards today.

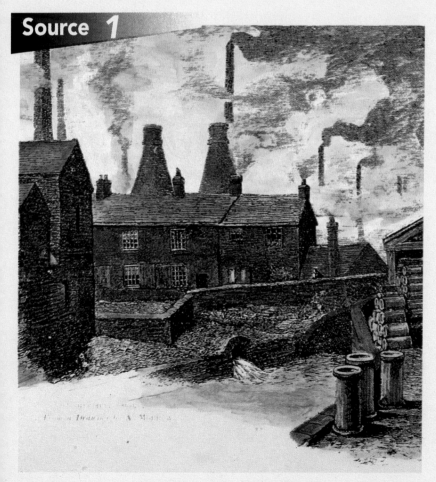

Source 1

▲ A view of industrial Sheffield in the mid-19th century.

One gruesome pollution problem was the disposal of dead bodies. Cremation was illegal until about 1850. Churchyards became overcrowded and posed a health threat, as this report on a London burial ground in the late 1830s shows:
The Portugal Street burial ground is truly shocking. It is crammed with coffins only two feet, in some places only fifteen inches below the surface. Yet the work of burials still goes on. The inhabitants of overlooking houses make dreadful complaints. Fever broods over the miserable place.

The problem was overcome by creating large public cemeteries on the outskirts of towns and cities.

CHAPTER 14

Conclusion

14.1 Change

Different rates of change

Medicine has not progressed steadily from prehistoric times until the present day.

Sometimes things changed quickly, sometimes not at all.

Sometimes things changed for the better, sometimes for the worse.

Also different aspects of medicine changed at different rates to others. We have studied these aspects of medicine:
- *ideas about the cause and cure of disease*
- *anatomy (how the human body works)*
- *surgery*
- *public health*
- *the medical profession (how the jobs of doctors and nurses developed).*

Graph A

Graph A shows one view of how the understanding of the **cause and cure of disease** varied through time. It shows how quickly things changed.

The fastest change is when the line is steep. Turning points probably happened at the points where there is a sharp change of angles.

Every 50 years has been given a mark out of 10 to suggest how much doctors knew at the time. These judgements were made to draw Graph A:

1 Understanding of cause and cure progressed rapidly in Greece at the time of Hippocrates.

2 From then, until the fall of the Roman Empire, there was slow but steady progress.

3 The was a sharp drop in understanding during the Dark Ages (regress).

4 Then, in the Middle Ages understanding began to rise slowly, speeding up after medical schools were set up.

5 There was rapid improvement during the Renaissance.

6 Then there was a gradual improvement until the mid-19th century when it was discovered that germs cause disease.

7 Since this discovery our knowledge about the cause and cure of disease has increased very rapidly.

Graph B

Graph B show how standards in **surgery** have changed over time. It has a pattern which is fairly similar to Graph A but it has a different time scale to Graph A. This is because we know a little about prehistoric surgery.

Comparing the graphs

There are other differences between the graphs. For example, between 1500 and 1800 understanding of the cause and cure of disease made more progress than surgery. But after 1800 it is surgery which improved more quickly, thanks to the development of **anaesthetics** and **antiseptics**.

Try to plot your own graphs for
- public health
- anatomy.

Think about the sorts of patterns they might follow. Would you expect them to be like Graph A, Graph B or neither?

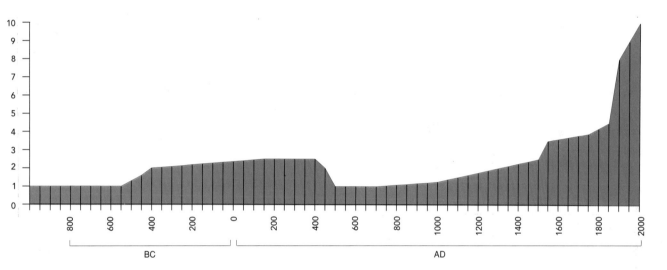

▲ **Graph A: Standards in understanding of the cause and cure of disease.**

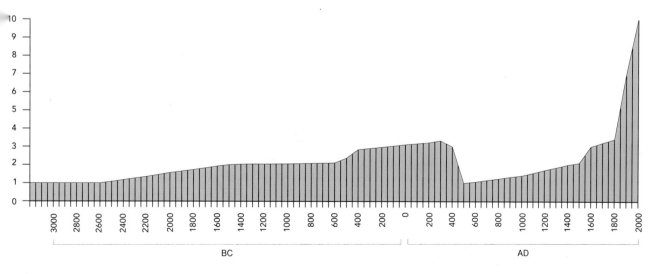

▲ **Graph B: Standards in surgery.**

• •

The suggestions for further reading given here include books that are not currently in print. However, they should be easily available, either because they are in the collections of many public libraries, or because they could always be ordered through the inter-library loan service. To make them easier to look up in library catalogues, or to order through inter-library loans, the original date of publication, rather than the most recent reprint has been given.

General histories

Ann G Carmichael and Richard M. Ratzen ed., *Medicine: A Treasury of Art and Literature*, Beaux Arts Editions, 1991. A combination of short extracts from primary sources, from historians, and a collection of pictures from early books and manuscripts. Very useful for illustrations.

Douglas Guthrie, *A History of Medicine*, Nelson, London, 1945. Covers from prehistoric times to the middle of the twentieth century. In many ways the best single volume history, well-written, illustrated, and giving a clear overview without missing out the detail which gives a flavour to the story.

Philip Rhodes, *An Outline History of Medicine*, Butterworths, London, 1985. An up to date summary with a useful chronology, though rather thin on medicine before the Renaissance.

Charles Singer and E. Asworth Underwood, *A Short History of Medicine*, second edition, Oxford University Press, 1962.

Much longer than Guthrie, with less on the civilizations before Greece, but clear and comprehensive.

Boswell Taylor, *How Things Developed: Medicine*, Ward Lock, London, 1965. One of the few texts written for school students. Rather simple and concentrating on a few major people and events.

Andrew Wear ed., *Medicine in Society: Historical Essays*, Cambridge University Press, 1992. A collection of essays rather than a comprehensive history, but with good modern summaries, especially of Greek and Roman medicine, and medieval medicine.

Specialist works

Lucinda McCray Beier, *Sufferers and Healers: The Experience of Illness in Seventeenth-Century England*, Routledge and Kegan Paul, London & New York, 1987. A complex academic monograph with a great deal of information about the experience of ordinary people when faced with disease and medicine. Full of quotations from primary sources.

W.J. Bishop, *The Early History of Surgery*, Robert Hale, London, 1961. A straightforward outline which spends time and space dealing with ancient and medieval surgery as well as Renaissance and later developments.

Ronald C. Finucane, *Miracles and Pilgrims: Popular Beliefs in Medieval England*, J.M. Dent and Sons, London, 1977. Concentrates on the miracle cults but with a lot of interesting information about the cures which were associated with them.

Geoffrey Keynes ed., *The Apologie and Treatise of Ambroise Pare*, Falcon Educational Books, London, 1951.
A useful introduction followed by the text of Paré's *Apologie* and selections from his other surgical writings.

G.E.R. Lloyd ed., *Hippocratic Writings*, Penguin, London, 1978.
A good modern translation of the most important of the Hippocratic books.

Norman Longmate, *Alive and Well: Medicine and Public Health 1830 to the Present Day*, Penguin, London, 1970.
Written for school students.

Jonathan Miller, *The Body in Question*, Jonathan Cape Ltd, London, 1978.
Not a history of medicine, but a book about the human body written to accompany a television series. Full of historical insights and especially good on the revolution in anatomy from Vesalius to Harvey.

Jurgen Thorwald, *The Century of the Surgeon*, Thames and Hudson, London, 1957.
A history of surgery from the mid 19th century written as if it were the memoirs of a man who had lived through the great changes described. A strange approach but one that covers a lot of information in an interesting way.

GLOSSARY

Abbasids a family which ruled the Muslim world from AD 750 to AD 1258.

anatomy the study of how the human skeleton is fitted together.

antibiotic a drug made from mould or fungus which kills many germs. Penicillin, discovered in 1928, was the first antibiotic.

antibodies a substance made in a person's blood which is able to fight infection.

antiseptic a substance which kills germs. The first antiseptic used in medicine was carbolic acid. Other antiseptics include chlorine and iodine.

archaeologist a person who digs up the ground looking for remains of the past such as buildings.

aseptic when an operating theatre is kept free of germs. This means sterilizing the air, tools and clothing of the surgeons.

'black period' of surgery a time between 1840 and 1870 when doctors carried out a lot of operations using anaesthetics. Many patients, however, died from infection because antiseptics had yet to come into use.

blood transfusions the replacement of lost blood during an operation. Doctors were unable to do successful transfusions until 1901 when it was found that there were four types of blood.

Board of Health a committee set up in some towns, usually after a cholera epidemic, to improve water supplies and drainage.

Buddhism a religion started in India in AD 528. It now has over 160 million followers.

cesspit a hole dug in the ground into which sewage was put.

chloroform a colourless chemical which was first used as a pain-killer, or anaesthetic, by James Simpson. It is no longer used as an anaesthetic.

Crusades a number of wars fought between Christians and Muslims, mainly in Palestine, during the Middle Ages.

Dark Ages the name given to the period of time between the fall of the Roman Empire in AD 410 and the Norman invasion of England in AD 1066. It was a time when a lot of books and learning was lost. Roman towns and buildings fell into ruin.

elements during ancient times and the Middle Ages many people thought that the planet was made up of four elements – earth, water, air and fire.

embalming preserving a dead body with chemicals.

empire a group of countries which are conquered and ruled by another well organized, powerful country.

ether a colourless chemical which was used as a pain-killer, or anaesthetic, during the 19th century.

Industrial Revolution the name given to the changes which turned Britain from a farming country to one of factories and large towns.

laissez-faire French for 'leave alone'. During the early 19th century people thought that the government should leave things like cleaning up towns to other people; it was not the job of the government to pass Acts to do this.

miasma a cloud of bad air. For a long time many people thought that disease was spread by bad air.

midwife a person who helps to deliver a baby.

mosque a place where Muslims worship.

Nobel Prize a prize given each year to people who do good work in medicine, science, literature and keeping the peace. This was the idea of a Swedish scientist called Alfred Nobel and was first awarded in 1901.

pilgrimage a journey to a holy place to worship. Pilgrimages were very common in the Middle Ages. For example, many pilgrims went to Canterbury to worship at the tomb of Thomas Becket.

prescription charges under the NHS people have to pay a charge to help towards the cost of medicine. Prescription charges were started in 1950.

rational something which is based on reason.

Reformation the movement to reform or change the Roman Catholic Church. The power of the Pope was questioned by people such as Martin Luther.

scarlet fever an illness mainly in children. Sufferers have a rash, high temperature and a sore throat.

transplant when a diseased part of the body, such as the heart, kidneys or liver, is cut away and replaced with a new part taken from another person.

typhoid a fever spread by a germ which lives in dirty water.

vaccination when a person is injected with a vaccine which gives protection against certain diseases. The first vaccination was against smallpox, discovered by Edward Jenner in 1796.